Sunshíne and Vítamín D

A Comprehensive Guide to the Benefits of the "Sunshine Vitamin"

Frank Murray

Foreword by Ronald L. Hoffman, MD

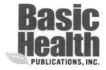

Basic Health
Health
PUBLICATIONS, INC.

The information contained in this book is based upon the research and personal and professional experiences of the author. It is not intended as a substitute for consulting with your physician or other healthcare provider. Any attempt to diagnose and treat an illness should be done under the direction of a healthcare professional.

The publisher does not advocate the use of any particular healthcare protocol but believes the information in this book should be available to the public. The publisher and author are not responsible for any adverse effects or consequences resulting from the use of the suggestions, preparations, or procedures discussed in this book. Should the reader have any questions concerning the appropriateness of any procedures or preparation mentioned, the author and the publisher strongly suggest consulting a professional healthcare advisor.

Vitamin D from the sun, diet, and supplements provides protection from osteoporosis, breast cancer, diabetes, gum disease, prostate cancer, multiple sclerosis, asthma, psoriasis, cystic fibrosis, colon cancer, celiac disease, osteoarthritis, Crohn's disease, scleroderma, rickets, osteomalacia, cardiovascular disease, and many other infirmities

Basic Health Publications, Inc.
28812 Top of the World Drive • Laguna Beach, CA 92651
949-715-7327 • www.basichealthpub.com

Library of Congress Cataloging-in-Publication Data

Murray, Frank.
    Sunshine and vitamin D / Frank Murray ; foreword by Ronald L. Hoffman.
       p. cm.
    Includes bibliographical references and index.
    ISBN 978-1-59120-250-9
  1. Vitamin D—Health aspects. 2. Sunshine—Health aspects. I. Title.

    QP772.V53M87   2008
    612.3'99—dc22

                                              2008028183

Editor: Diana Drew
Typesetting/Book design: Gary A. Rosenberg
Cover design: Mike Stromberg

Printed in the United States of America

10   9   8   7   6   5   4   3   2   1

Contents

Foreword

Vitamin D is hot! The vitamin D story is emblematic of how conventional medicine resists nutritional innovation. During my twenty-five-year career, I have seen a stunning reversal in medicine's attitude toward this potent therapeutic agent. It went from pariah—widely accused of being "toxic"—to grudging acknowledgment, and now, finally, it claims its rightful, preeminent place in the pantheon of vitamins.

When RDAs for vitamin D were established, they were set arbitrarily, based on the amount of vitamin D that could be found in a teaspoon of cod-liver oil, the traditional antidote to rickets. It has only recently been discovered that this level of fortification is insufficient to stave off diseases like osteoporosis, cancer, autoimmune conditions, and a host of health woes, as Frank Murray has pointed-ed out so eloquently in his groundbreaking book.

Moreover, we have compounded the problem by undertaking an irrational campaign against sun exposure, spearheaded by dermatologists and cancer organizations. Inadvertently, this has magnified the epidemic of vitamin D deficiency that affects Western countries.

It is only due to the efforts of a few stalwart scientists that we have pierced the veil of ignorance surrounding vitamin D. Dr. Michael Holick earned the derision of his colleagues merely by having the temerity to suggest that "healthy tanning" was not an oxymoron. But he was vindicated when, in 2007, he was invited to author a prominent review article in the mainstream *New England Journal of Medicine,* which boldly advocated higher doses of vitamin D and moderate sun exposure.

Dr. John Cannell, champion of the Vitamin D Council, also sowed controversy whenever he lectured to medical professionals. In an interview on my radio program, *Health Talk,* he revealed that he used to leave his audiences aghast after stepping to the podium and promptly downing an entire bottle of vitamin D capsules to underscore the vitamin's lack of toxicity (don't try this at home!).

Now come new indications that vitamin D, in addition to preventing many diseases and ameliorating others, may have the ability to extend longevity itself. The "bone vitamin" has suddenly morphed into a virtual nutritional panacea!

So irresistible is the tide of new information about vitamin D that the public has embraced it in advance of the majority of health professionals. That is no coincidence: the vitamin D story exemplifies the populist revolution in health care that is sweeping the country, as more and more people gravitate toward natural alternatives, eschewing more risky and expensive medical interventions. The hidebound medical establishment often has a lag time of ten to fifteen years in accepting innovation. Belated mainstreaming of omega-3 fatty acids from fish, low-carb diets, and mind/body medicine are but a few examples.

I first began testing patients for vitamin D levels fifteen years ago, when it was considered medically unorthodox. In 1997, in my book *Intelligent Medicine,* I called for mandatory screening for vitamin D. Then in 2005 I made it part of my recommended physical in *How to Talk to Your Doctor.* All my patients at the Hoffman Center are now tested for vitamin D. It has been exciting for me to be on the cusp of the vitamin D paradigm shift, and now I see my faith in its therapeutic use vindicated by new studies and mainstream acceptance. As a clinician, I can verify that Frank Murray's perspective is accurate.

With the new and exciting information in *Sunshine and Vitamin D,* the public stands to be empowered with a key wellness tool. The fortunate readers of this book will be ahead of the curve on this, one of the most exciting health stories of the twenty-first century.

—Ronald L. Hoffman, MD
Host of *Health Talk*
www.drhoffman.com
New York City

Introduction

With the hundreds of clinical trials published on vitamin D in recent years—I read one study with 132 references—it is obvious that the "sunshine vitamin" no longer has to play second fiddle to the other vitamins. However, some of the currently available health books either ignore the vitamin or give it short shrift in just a few paragraphs. This has prompted several internationally respected scientists to call vitamin D the most misunderstood and underrated vitamin of all. To muddy the waters still further, other researchers insist that it is a hormone rather than a vitamin. In the meantime, millions of people around the world have a vitamin D deficiency, costing them lots of money, pain, and poor health.

Now that the vitamin has become a superstar, one wonders why it took so long for it to be recognized. As an example, how many life-threatening illnesses might be prevented with vitamin D? To paraphrase Elizabeth Barrett Browning, let us count the ways: osteoporosis, breast cancer, psoriasis, asthma, prostate cancer, multiple sclerosis, osteoarthritis, cardiovascular disease, diabetes, gum disease, colon cancer, Crohn's disease, scleroderma, rickets, celiac disease, and many others. How many other vitamins—say vitamin B_2—have such an impressive résumé? Not many!

When people moved away from the equator and settled in higher latitudes, they lost many of the life-nourishing benefits of the sun—a major source of vitamin D. To compound the problem, the vitamin is only available in a few foods. For example, how many of the following staples are on your grocery list—salmon, cod, eel, sardines, cod-liver oil, and beef liver? Fortunately, in the United States a quart of milk contains 400 IU of the vitamin. The fly in the ointment is that many seniors, young girls, and those who are lactose-intolerant do not drink milk regularly.

1

1.

The Sunshine Vitamin

Little is known about when vitamin D made its appearance on earth and what its function was, reported Michael F. Holick, MD, of Boston University School of Medicine in Massachusetts. However, it is known that some of the earliest phytoplankton and diatom life forms produced ergosterol (previtamin D_2).[1] This includes *Emiliania huxlei*, which had existed in the oceans for over 750 million years and which had used calcium for its structural support.

"When exposed to simulated sunlight, the ergosterol in E. huxlei was converted to previtamin D_2, which rapidly isomerized to vitamin D_2," Holick said. "*Skeletonema menzelii*, a diatom that also contained ergosterol, converted it to previtamin D_2."

He added that little is known about the biological function of ergosterol, previtamin D_2, and vitamin D_2 in convertebral species; however, it has been suggested that ergosterol and its photoproducts are an ideal sunscreening system because of their high absorption of ultraviolet radiation. Ergosterol, previtamin D_2, vitamin D_2, and their photoproducts efficiently absorb the UV radiation that is damaging to DNA, RNA, and protein.

"Thus, before the ozone layer—which now efficiently absorbs all UV radiation—evolved, the ergosterol-vitamin D_2 system may have played a critical role in protecting organisms from the high energy UV radiation that could have damaged their UV sensitive proteins, RNA, and DNA," Holick continued. "It is also possible that, if ergosterol existed in the plasma membrane of early life forms, it altered the membrane's permeability for calcium when it was converted to the structurally less rigid vitamin D_2."

In his concise article, Robert P. Heaney puts into perspective the many health benefits of vitamin D and the role of vitamin D deficiency in increasing the risk of many common and serious diseases, including some common cancers, type 1 diabetes, cardiovascular disease, and osteoporosis.[2]

"I have provided guidelines for the amount of sun exposure needed by people of all skin types to achieve their vitamin D requirement without significantly increasing the risk of skin damage and skin cancer," Heaney continued. "Increasingly, the intakes of food fortified with vitamin D, including milk, orange juice, cereals, and oily fish, is a reasonable approach satisfying the body's requirement. Taking over one multivitamin is counterproductive, since too much vitamin A could be ingested, and this increases the risk of birth defects and osteoporosis. Alternatively, one multivitamin containing 400 IU of vitamin D and a vitamin D supplement containing either 400 or 1,000 IU of vitamin D is appropriate."

The importance of vitamin D—the sunshine vitamin—in human nutrition lies in its role of regulating calcium and phosphorus metabolism, according to the *Foods & Nutrition Encyclopedia*. The vitamin promotes intestinal absorption of the two minerals and it influences the process of bone mineralization. Without vitamin D, mineralization in bone matrix is impaired, which results in rickets in children and osteomalacia in adults.[3]

A bone disorder, which we now call rickets, has been known since 500 B.C., but the disease was first properly described in London about three hundred years ago. The word *rickets* is derived from the Old English word *wrikken,* meaning "to bend or twist."

"Vitamin D is unique among vitamins in two respects: (1) it occurs naturally in only a few foods—mainly in fish oils and a little in liver, eggs, and milk—and (2) it can be formed in the body by exposure of the skin to ultraviolet rays of the sun—light of short wavelength and high frequency, hence, it is known as the 'sunshine vitamin,'" the encyclopedia reported.

During the Industrial Revolution in England in the eighteenth century, rickets became very prevalent in children in the crowded slums. Industrial smoke and high tenement buildings shut out the sunlight. Therefore, as industrial cities grew, rickets spread. Little was known about the sunshine connection, and rickets was blamed on bad home environment and poor hygiene, leading doctors to brand the condition as "a disease of poverty and darkness."

In 1824, the *Encyclopedia* continued, cod-liver oil, long known as a folk medicine, was found to be an important treatment for rickets. However, the treatment lost favor with the medical profession because doctors could not explain how it worked.

In 1890, Dr. Palm, an English physician, observed that when sunshine was abundant, rickets was rare. In 1918, Sir Edward Mellanby of England, demonstrated that rickets was a nutritional deficiency disease. He produced rickets in puppies and then cured them with cod-liver oil. However, he mistakenly attributed the cure to the newly discovered fat-soluble vitamin A.

"In 1922, E. V. McCollum at Johns Hopkins University, Baltimore, Maryland, found that, after destruction of all of the vitamin A in cod-liver oil—oxidation, bypassing heated air through cod-liver oil—it still retained its rickets-preventing potency," the *Encyclopedia* added. "This proved the existence of a second fat-soluble vitamin, carried in liver oils and certain other fats, which he called 'calcium-depositing vitamin.' While McCollum discovered vitamin D, he did not call it that until after this designation was in common use by others."

In 1924, the mystery of how sunlight could prevent rickets was partially solved by Harry Steenbock, MD, of the University of Wisconsin and A. Hess, MD, of Columbia University in New York, who, while working independently, found that antirachitic activity could be produced in foods and in animals by ultraviolet light. This process, known as the Steenbock Irradiation Process, was patented in his name.

By the 1920s, it had been concluded that rickets could be prevented and cured by exposure to direct sunlight, by irradiation with ultraviolet light, by eating irradiated food, or by consuming cod-liver oil. Later, the vitamin D of fish liver oils was identified as the same substance that is produced in the skin by irradiation, the *Encyclopedia* said.

"In 1932, crystals of pure vitamin D_2 (ergocalciferol) were isolated from irradiated ergosterol by Adolf Otto Reinhold Windaus (1876–1959), a German chemist, and Dr. Askew in England; and, in 1936, crystals of pure vitamin D_3 (cholecalciferol) were isolated from tuna liver oil by a Dr. Brockmann in Germany. In 1952, the first total synthesis of a form of vitamin D (vitamin D_3) was accomplished by R. B. Woodward of Harvard University, for which he received the Nobel Prize in chemistry in 1965," the *Encyclopedia* continued. (Ergosterol is a crystalline sterol alcohol in yeast, molds, and ergot [fungi], which is converted by UV irradiation into vitamin D_2.)

Although about ten sterol components with vitamin D activity have been isolated, only two—known as provitamins D or precursors—are of practical importance from the standpoint of their occurrence in foods: ergocalciferol (vitamin D_2, calciferol, or viosterol) and cholecalciferol (vitamin D_3). Cholecalciferol is a reflection of its cholesterol precursor. Since these substances are so closely related chemically, the term *vitamin D* is used collectively to indicate the group that shows this vitamin activity, the publication said.

Ultraviolet irradiation of ergosterol and 7-dehydrocholesterol will produce vitamin D_2 and vitamin D_3, respectively. Ergosterol is found in plants, whereas vitamin D_3 is available in fish liver oils and in the skin. Vitamin D_2 and vitamin D_3 have comparable efficacy in combating disease.

"When the skin is exposed to the UV radiation of sunlight, part of the store of 7-dehydrocholesterol undergoes a photochemical reaction in the epidermis and the dermis and forms previtamin D_3," the publication added. "Once previtamin D_3 is formed in the skin, it undergoes a slow temperature-dependent transformation to vitamin D_3, which takes about 3 days to complete. Then, the vitamin D-binding protein transports vitamin D_3 from the skin into circulation."

Cholecalciferol, either from the diet or from irradiation of the skin, is transported by a vitamin D carrier protein (a globulin) to the liver, where it is converted into 25-hydroxycholecalciferol—$25(OH)D_3$. From the liver, this substance is transported to the kidneys, where it is converted to $1,25\text{-}(OH)_2D_3$, the most active form of vitamin D in increasing calcium absorption, bone calcium mobilization, and increased intestinal phosphate absorption.

The *Encyclopedia* goes on to say that the active compound—$1,25\text{-}(OH)_2D_3$—functions as a hormone, since it is a necessary substance made in the body tissues (the kidneys) and transported in the blood to cells within target tissues. The physiological active form of vitamin D_3 is then either moved to its various sites or converted to its metabolite forms—24,25-dihydroxycholecalciferol or 1,24,25-trihydroxycholecalciferol.

While most of the research on vitamin D metabolism has been conducted on cholecalciferol, studies by Dr. DeLuca on ergocalciferol suggest that it is metabolized similarly to cholecalciferol and that it is changed to a similar active metabolite in the liver—25 hydroxy-ergocalciferol, or $25(OH)D_2$.

Vitamin D potency is expressed in international units (IU) and U.S. pharmacopoeia units (USP), which are equivalent, added the *Encyclopedia*. One IU or one USP of vitamin D is defined as the activity of 0.025 mcg of pure crystalline vitamin D_3 (cholecalciferol). The UV light absorption property of vitamin D may be used for the assay of pure preparations free of irrelevant absorption. However, it does not distinguish between vitamin D_2 and vitamin D_3.

"The principal storage sites of vitamin D are the fatty tissues and skeletal muscle," the *Encyclopedia* said. "Some of it is also found in the liver, brain, lungs, spleen, bones, and skin. However, body stores of vitamin D are more limited than the storage of fat-soluble vitamin A."

Vitamin D increases calcium absorption from the small intestine, and a vitamin D deficiency produces large losses of calcium in the feces. Sufficient vitamin D enhances the levels of phosphates in the body because of: (1) improved absorption of phosphorus through the intestinal wall, independent of calcium absorption; and (2) increased resorption of phosphates from the kidney tubules. When sufficient amounts of vitamin D are not available, urinary excretion of phosphate increases and the blood level drops, the publication added.

Vitamin D deficiency is characterized by inadequate mineralization of the bone, according to *Recommended Dietary Allowances,* a publication of the Food and Nutrition Board of the National Research Council in Washington, D.C. In children, severe deficiency leads to deformation of the skeleton, or rickets. In adults, a vitamin D deficiency results in undermineralization of the bone matrix osteoid. This results in hypocalcemia, which is accompanied by secondary hyperthyroidism that leads to excessive bone loss and, in extreme cases, bone fractures or osteomalacia. The prolonged time required to produce a vitamin D deficiency is attributed to the gradual release of vitamin D–related steroids from fat deposits and the skin.[4]

"Since milk and other foods are fortified with vitamin D, rickets is rare in many countries; however, a vitamin D deficiency occurs in some infants who are breastfed without supplemental vitamin D or exposure to sunlight, the elderly, as well as in those with vitamin D malabsorption," the publication added. "Abnormalities in calcium balance and bone metabolism can also occur when the conversion of vitamin D to biologically active forms is compromised by disease. As an example, rickets and osteomalacia are often found in patients with kidney failure."

Vitamin D status is reflected in the concentrations of 25(OH)D and 1,25(OH)$_2$D in the blood, the publication continued. In surveys of healthy people, the mean value of 25(OH)D ranges from about 25 to 30 ng/ml. The concentrations of 1,25(OH)$_2$D range from 18 to 60 pg/ml of plasma in normal children and between 15 and 45 pg/ml in healthy adults. Pg stands for picogram, which is one-trillionth of a gram. Ng stands for nanogram, or one-billionth of a gram.

Processed cow's milk, which contains 10 mcg of cholecalciferol (400 IU) per quart, contributes most of the vitamin ingested by children, the publication said. Infant formulas are fortified with the same amount as milk. Human milk contains 0.63 to 1.25 mcg of cholecalciferol per liter.

At its birth almost a century ago, nutritional science had to overcome the prevailing view that all disease was caused by external invaders, either bacterial or toxic, explained Robert P. Heaney, MD, of Creighton University in Omaha, Nebraska. He added that we owe much to pioneers like E. V. McCollum, who were convinced—and ultimately convinced the scientific and medical communities—that foods contained substances the body needs for good health, and that not getting enough of them caused disease.[5]

"Unfortunately, the medical community's approach to nutrition is still strongly influenced by the early external invader model," Heaney added. "Some of the most prominent contemporary medical nutritional efforts, such as those involving cholesterol, saturated fat, and salt, typify that paradigm. Additionally, scarcely a day passes without finding a report in the general news media or a study linking this or that cancer—or other dire outcome—with consumption of some nutrient. Clearly, the toxicity model continues to capture the attention of the medical community."

He goes on to say that rickets/osteomalacia is generally thought to be brought on by malabsorption of calcium and phosphorus and that this is correct, as far as it goes. As the efficiency of calcium absorption decreases, parathyroid hormone (PTH) secretion increases. The latter stimulates synthesis of calcitriol, which improves calcium absorption efficiency, but evidently not enough to make up the difference, thus leading to still further increases in PTH concentration.

At the same time, he continued, PTH concentrations lower the kidney threshold for phosphorus, which, together with reduced phosphorus absorption, produces hyperphosphatemia. It is this development that impairs osteoblast and chondroblast cell function and leads to disordered metaphysical growth plates and the characteristic histologic features of rickets and osteomalacia.

"The modest vitamin D fortification of milk and other foods, coupled with the use of vitamin D supplements in children, has eliminated most cases of Stage 3 vitamin D deficiency in North America," Heaney said. "However, these same stratagems have not been sufficient to prevent the lesser degree of deficiency. The vitamin D supplements are pegged to the prevention of Stage 3 deficiency and there still remains a presumption that if one does not have rickets or osteomalacia, then they have sufficient vitamin D."

Only recently have reliable measurements of serum 25(OH)D concentrations been available, and most of the physiology of vitamin D has been worked out before that time and, thus, was unconnected to specific levels of vitamin D repletion, Heaney added. As an example, the Food and Nutrition Board had no difficulty in identifying 25(OH)D as the functional indicator for vitamin D status, but the Board was not able, with the data then available, to assign numerical values to the lower limit of the normal range, or to assign cutoff values for various vitamin D activities.

"As a result," he said, "current recommendations are usually related to laboratory 'reference' ranges—which are inevitably circular, inasmuch as such ranges record what is observed in people who are considered 'normal' only because they do not have rickets or osteomalacia. A large body of data relating to parathyroid hormone to circulating 25(OH)D concentrations indicate that the lower end of an acceptable normal range must be about 80 nmol/l. By contrast, the lower end of most reference ranges is closer to 40 nmol/l."

Nutritional scientists often refer to values less than 20 nmol/l as "deficient," since they were reproducibly associated with osteomalacia or rickets, and values above around 80 nmol/l as "normal." Values in between are considered "insufficient," without a clear consensus as to where the boundary might lie between "insufficient" and "normal," Heaney added.

Concerning calcium economy, it now appears that scientific studies, at least for those in North America and the United Kingdom, indicate values below 80 nmol/l are deficient, he said.

"The awkward term *insufficiency* ought to be dropped," he added. "It's use simply reflected by the usual observations that the index disease for vitamin D was osteomalacia and rickets. If one had it, they were *deficient* and if they did not, one could not be *deficient.*"

In the 1999 issue of *Clinical Pearls,* Kirk Hamilton, PA.C., interviewed Reinhold Vieth, PhD, of Mt. Sinai Hospital in Toronto, who stated that vitamin D is perhaps the most misunderstood and underrated of vitamins.[6]

In some ways, vitamin D is like cholesterol, Vieth explained, in that cholesterol is the raw material for making steroid hormones, including sex hormones and cortisol. However, unlike cholesterol, the amount of vitamin D available for hormone production is minute and arbitrary, mostly dependent on UV-B exposure and, to a lesser degree, upon dietary intake.

Vieth goes on to say there are several cancers whose prevalence increases as one heads north in latitude, especially breast, ovarian, and prostate cancers. And multiple sclerosis is more common in regions with less ultraviolet light.

Based on objective, measurable criteria, vitamin D deficiency is by far the most common nutritional deficiency in northern latitudes, especially in those over sixty years of age, Vieth added.

"In the winter, half of the people on my hospital's laboratory staff fall into the insufficient vitamin D category," Vieth said. "This situation is at least as bad in the elderly."

He added that it is his contention that vitamin D is not a natural part of the human diet, since it is not present in plants normally consumed by humans and that the best dietary sources are fatty fish like salmon, cod, or halibut. Most of the vitamin D we get from foods was artificially added. As an example, there is essentially no vitamin D naturally present in milk.

Exposure of most of the skin of an adult to a nonburning amount of UV light—fifteen minutes of summer sun for a white person—provides at least 10,000 IUs of vitamin D, Vieth continued. However, since the skin of those over sixty-five produces less cholesterol—necessary for the conversion to vitamin D—the same sunshine results in only about one-third the amount of vitamin D as would be available to a younger person. In addition, as the sun sits lower in the sky during winter months, there is not enough UV radiation in the light that reaches the earth to generate vitamin D.

He added that people with bone disease should be tested for serum 25(OH)D levels, but he insists that our nutritional guidelines concerning vitamin D are way out of whack for adults. Cod-liver oil has been used for some two hundred years to prevent rickets in infants, and in adults, 200 IU RDA is equivalent to half a teaspoon of cod-liver oil. The adult intake was set arbitrarily, and it does not stand up to any critical scrutiny.

When asked about side effects of high doses of vitamin D, Vieth said that severe cases—that is, consuming more than 40,000 IU/day for many months—cause circulating calcium levels to increase. This amount produces constipation, excessive urination, reduced reflexes, and higher calcium in the urine. However, he added, he would contend that the more harmful situation relates to the side effects of too low a level of vitamin D nutrition.

At Boston University Medical Center in Massachusetts, Michael F. Holick, MD, and his colleagues did a study involving young adults, eighteen to twenty-nine years of age, in the Boston area, and found that 36 percent were deficient in vitamin D at the end of winter. And they were 11 percent deficient at the end of summer.[7]

Holick added that you can store fat-soluble vitamin D in body fat, assuming that you get enough of the vitamin with adequate exposure to sunlight in spring, summer, and fall. The vitamin will later be released during the winter. It is, therefore, important for those who live in northern areas and those who spend most of their time indoors, to get outdoors so their bodies can make and store adequate vitamin D.

"We and others have shown over and over that older adults are prone to vitamin D deficiency," Holick continued. "A study in Baltimore showed that up to 50 and 60 percent of free-living adults over the age of 65 were severely vitamin D deficient."

What about sunshine and skin cancer? Holick advises spending five to fifteen minutes in the sun to get your vitamin D and then go inside and apply a sunscreen with SPF 15 to protect against sun damage before going outside again.

Does this apply to all skin conditions? He said that depends on the person and his sensitivity to sunlight. For example, new research suggests that African Americans may require more time outdoors to produce enough vitamin D. He estimated that up to 40 percent of African Americans in the Boston area are deficient in the vitamin.

In the same issue of the *New York Times,* Bill Marsh reported that long hours indoors and heavy use of sunscreens leaves some people deficient in vitamin D, even in the summer. As an example, a sunscreen with an SPF of 8 blocks 97.5 percent of vitamin D–making rays.[8]

How long can you be in the sun without burning? Marsh suggested dividing this time by four—sunburn in sixty minutes divided by four equals fifteen minutes. Exposure to that much sun on the face and hands two or three times weekly—except in the winter—should be adequate.

There is now a consensus that serum 25-hydroxyvitamin D—25(OH)D—concentration is the correct functional indicator, but what is less certain is what the optimal concentration of 25(OH)D should be and how much we must produce or ingest to achieve it, reported Robert P. Heaney, MD, in the *American Journal of Clinical Nutrition.*[9]

He added that A. M. Parfitt, building on the expansion of knowledge in bone biology, has characterized the disorder due to insufficient vitamin D as "hypovitaminosis D osteopathy" (HVO). Parfitt divides HVO into three stages along a scale of increasing severity. In Stage 1 HVO, there is malabsorption of calcium accompanied by physiologic evidence of an attempt to compensate—for example, elevated parathyroid hormone production and high bone remodeling. The result is bone loss or osteoporosis.[10]

"In Stage 2 HVO, bone mass is also low, calcium malabsorption continues, and bone remodeling is either high or drops back into the normal range and histologic examination of bone reveals sub-clinical, early osteomalacia," Heaney added. "In Stage 3 HVO, clinical rickets or osteomalacia is present and bone remodeling is reduced or absent—partly because of the dependence of bone resorption on 1,25-dihydroxyvitamin D (1,25(OH)D) and partly because bony surfaces covered with unmineralized osteoid serve as barriers to osteoclastic erosion."

As Reinhold Vieth has reported, Heaney continued, total daily intake, production, or both amount to 2.5 to 5 mcg (100–200 IU) of vitamin D and serum 25(OH)D concentrations—over 20 to 25 nmol/l—sufficient to prevent Stage 3 HVO.[11]

"However, the mere absence of clinical rickets can hardly be considered an adequate definition either of health or of vitamin D sufficiency," Heaney continued. "This is especially important in view of the worldwide evidence of osteoporosis, which, although a multifactorial disorder like high blood pressure and coronary artery disease, can, nevertheless, also be produced by milder degrees of vitamin D insufficiency, that is Stages 1 and 2 HVO."

Current studies to assess optimum serum concentrations of 25-hydroxyvitamin D generally focus on bone health in older white people, and the common definition of the optimal vitamin D concentrations has been the concentrations that maximally suppress serum parathyroid hormone, reported Heike A. Bischoff-Ferrari of the Harvard School of Public Health, Boston, Massachusetts and colleagues in the United States and Switzerland.[12, 13, 14]

"This is a useful criterion since parathyroid hormone promotes bone loss, but fluctuations related to diet, time of day, kidney function, and physical activity raise concerns with respect to this approach," Bischoff-Ferrari and colleagues said. "Estimates of optimal vitamin D concentrations reached by using the parathyroid hormone criterion vary widely, from 20 to 110 nmol/l (9 to 38 ng/ml) and a consensus has not been reached. Blood levels of vitamin D have also been related to calcium absorption, but these studies did not allow for estimation of a precise threshold."

The review by Bischoff-Ferrari and colleagues summarizes evidence from studies that evaluated thresholds of serum 25(OH)D concentrations relating to bone mineral density, a lower extremity function, dental health, and risk of falls, fractures, and colorectal cancer. For all endpoints, the most advantageous serum concentrations of vitamin D begin at 75 nmol/l (30 ng/ml), and the best are between 90 and 100 nmol/l (36 to 40 ng/ml), the researchers said.

"In most people, these concentrations could not be reached with the currently recommended intakes of 200 to 600 IU/day of vitamin D for younger and older adults, respectively," the researchers continued. "A comparison of vitamin D intakes with achieved serum concentrations of 25(OH)D for the purpose of estimating optimal intakes led us to suggest that for bone health in younger adults and all studied outcomes in older adults, an increase in the currently recommended intake of vitamin D is warranted."

In evaluating patients who are deficient in vitamin D, just how much of the vitamin do they actually need? As reported in the *New England Journal of Medicine,* Melissa K. Thomas, MD, PhD, and colleagues at Massachusetts General Hospital in Boston evaluated 164 patients who were considered to be vitamin D–deficient, with a blood level of 25-hydroxyvitamin D of less than or equal to 15 ng/ml. Twenty-two percent were said to be severely vitamin D–deficient, with levels less than 8 ng/ml.[15]

Thomas added that blood levels of 25-hydroxyvitamin D were inversely related to parathyroid hormone concentrations. In fact, 66 percent of the patients who consumed less than the recommended daily amount of the vitamin, and 37 percent of those with intakes above the recommended daily amount, were vitamin D–deficient.

As often reported, a vitamin D deficiency is associated with muscle weakness, and this is common in elderly people, according to Hennie C. J. P. Janssen of the University Medical Center, Utrecht, Netherlands, and a research team at the same institution. The gradual loss of muscle strength—below a certain threshold—results in functional impairment, the need for assistance in the performance of daily activities, and an increased risk of falling as well as nonvertebral fractures.[16, 17, 18]

A vitamin D deficiency is common in the elderly because of various risk factors, such as decreased dietary intake, diminished sunlight exposure, reduced skin thickness, impaired intestinal absorption, and impaired hydroxylation in the liver and kidneys, the researchers said.

They added that, of 824 elderly people over seventy years of age from eleven European countries, 36 percent of the men and 47 percent of the women had wintertime blood levels of 25-hydroxyvitamin D_3 concentrations less than 30 nmol/l.

"From experimental studies, it was found that vitamin D metabolites directly influence muscle cell maturation and functioning through a vitamin D receptor," added Janssen and colleagues. "Vitamin D supplementation in vitamin D deficient, elderly people improved muscle strength, walking distance, and functional ability and resulted in a reduction in falls and non-vertebral fractures."

Vitamin D insufficiency in adults causes myopathy, osteopenia, secondary hyperthyroidism, and osteomalacia, reported Mark J. Bolland of the University of Auckland, New Zealand, and colleagues at other locations. In their study, they set out to determine the effects of seasonal variation of 25(OH)D on a previously selected minimum concentration for vitamin D sufficiency (50 nmol/l) and to determine whether fat mass modifies these effects.[19]

The study evaluated 1,606 healthy postmenopausal women and 378 older men from Auckland who were undergoing measurements of 25(OH)D.

The researchers found that concentrations of less than 50 nmol/l of vitamin D were seen in 49 percent of the women and 9 percent of the men, and 73 percent of the women and 39 percent of the men were found to have vitamin D concentrations of less than 50 nmol/l, according to seasonal variations.

The researchers said that seasonal variations significantly affect the diagnosis of vitamin D sufficiency, which requires seasonally adjusted thresholds, individualized for different locations. Therefore, clinicians should consider the month of sampling and the amount of body fat when interpreting 25(OH)D measurements.

Ecological and observational studies suggest that low vitamin D intake could be associated with higher mortality from life-threatening conditions, such as cancer, cardiovascular disease, and diabetes mellitus, which account for 60–70 percent of total mortality in high-income countries, reported *Archives of Internal Medicine*. The study examined the risk of dying from any cause in those who participated in studies involving vitamin D and health.[20]

The medical literature in all languages was searched up to November 2006 and the researchers identified eighteen independent, randomized, controlled trials, involving 57,311 people. A total of 4,777 deaths from any cause occurred during the five- to seven-year period. Daily vitamin doses ranged from 300 to 2,000 IU, with the mean intake being 528 IU. The addition of calcium did not influence the outcome.

The researchers reported that intake of ordinary doses of vitamin D supplements seemed to be associated with decreased total mortality rates. They suggested that placebo-controlled, randomized trials should confirm these findings.

The use of dietary supplements could offer health benefits, as well as save the United States over $24 billion in health care costs over the next five years, according to a survey by the Lewin Group in 2004 and 2005. The survey was commissioned by the Dietary Supplement Education Alliance in Sarasota, Florida.[21]

The study reported that, if those with Medicare benefits used appropriate doses of calcium and vitamin D, almost 776,000 hospitalizations for hip fractures would be avoided over five years. Reducing these hospital stays would save an estimated $16.1 billion.

A research team at the Jean Meyer/U.S. Department of Agriculture Human Nutrition Research Center on Aging at Tufts University in Boston and other facilities, headed by Paul F. Jacques, PhD, conducted a study involving 290 men and 469 women, ranging in age from sixty-seven to ninety-five, which confirmed that elderly people who took a vitamin supplement or drank two to three glasses of milk daily had sufficient vitamin D levels in their blood. However, 75 percent of the women and 80 percent of the men did not regularly take vitamin supplements, and among this group 68 percent of the women and 64 percent of the men consumed less than eight ounces (227g) of milk daily.[22]

Arthur A. Knapp, MD, a New York ophthalmologist, treated some of his older eye patients with massive doses of vitamin D, reported Ruth Adams. He believed that myopia or shortsightedness is not just an eye condition, but is instead a manifestation of a vitamin D deficiency.[23]

Knapp gave a group of his patients vitamin D and calcium supplements from five to twenty-eight months and found a decrease in nearsightedness in more than one-third of them, with a definite halt in the progress toward nearsightedness in another 17 percent. He discussed his protocol at a 1966 meeting of the American Geriatrics Society.

"Knapp almost believed that a lack of vitamin D and calcium may be related to the formation of cataracts, although he admitted that not enough research has been done along these lines," Adams added. "He said that laboratory animals kept on diets deficient in vitamin D and calcium invariably developed cataracts."

Researchers at the Minerva Foundation Institute for Medical Research in Helsinki, Finland, evaluated vegetarians, lacto-vegetarians, and lacto-ovo-vegetarians and found that strict vegetarians were especially low in vitamin D. Finnish patients were particularly vulnerable because of Finland's northern latitude in the winter months, when sunlight is at a minimum.[24]

There are several case reports in the literature suggesting that infants developed cataracts because their mothers were deficient in vitamin D, according to the *Lancet.*[25]

Researchers at the Veterans Affairs Medical Center, Bronx, New York, evaluated fifty patients with spinal cord injuries and fifty controls without an injury and found that almost one-third of the spinal cord injury patients were deficient in vitamin D.[26]

It was reported that some of the patients exhibited mild, secondary, hyper-parathyroidism and abnormally low levels of calcium circulating in their blood. The researchers suggested that these patients should be treated with adequate amounts of vitamin D and calcium supplements, reported *Metabolism.*

In noninstitutionalized children with cerebral palsy, there is a high preva-lence of low blood levels of calcidiol (25-hydroxycholecalciferol), especially in the winter, according to Richard C. Henderson, MD, PhD, in the *Journal of Child Neurology.*[27]

The prevalence of low levels of calcidiol—less than 10 ng/dl—was found in 19 percent of the patients. Less than 2 percent of the children were found to have a low level of calcidiol—less than 20 ng/dl.

Vitamin D supplements during pregnancy could improve bone health and reduce the risk of osteoporotic fractures in a woman's offspring, according to a British research study (M. K. Javaid et al., "Maternal Vitamin D Status during Pregnancy and Childhood Bone Mass at Age 9 Years: A Longitudinal Study," *Lancet* 367 [2006]: 36–43), reported Joan Stephenson, PhD, in the *Journal of the American Medical Association.*[28]

In a logitudinal study involving 198 children born in 1991 and 1992, the research team found that those born to mothers with deficient levels of vitamin D—less than 11 mcg/l—had significantly lower whole body and lumbar spine bone mineral content at nine years of age, compared with those whose moth-ers were "vitamin D replete"—over 20 mcg/l. Children whose mothers took vitamin D supplements and those born during summer months had significant-ly higher bone mineral density.

Stephenson added that, "Vitamin D insufficiency was a frequent finding in this group of white women. However, vitamin supplementation, especially when the last trimester of pregnancy occurs during the winter, could lead to an enhanced peak bone mineral accrual and a reduced risk of fragility fracture in offspring during later life."

An article by Mary E. Mohs, PhD, RD, in the *Journal of the American Dietet-ic Association,* reviewed the nutritional effects of the use of marijuana, heroin, cocaine, and nicotine. These addictive substances can affect food and liquid intake behavior, taste preferences, and body weight.[29]

Heroin addiction can cause hyperkalemia (abnormal amounts of potassium in the blood) and morphine can result in calcium inhibition, Mohs said. Morphine also causes hypercholesterolemia (abnormal amounts of cholesterol in the blood), hypothermia (low body temperature), and hyperthermia (high fever).

In addition, she said, diabetes decreases sensitivity to and dependence on morphine, protein deprivation produces preferential fat utilization, and low cocaine use and vitamin D deficiency decelerates morphine dependency.

A study headed by Robert N. Davidson, MD, and colleagues, reported in the *Lancet,* found that 25-hydroxycholecalciferol deficiency may contribute to the high incidence of tuberculosis in an immigrant population originally from Gujarat, a region in western India. The participants were mainly vegetarians with TB.[30]

The research team evaluated blood levels of 25-hydroxycholecalciferol in 103 patients and 42 controls. It was found that 25-hydroxycholecalciferol deficiency was associated with active TB, and undetectable serum 25-hydroxycholecalciferol carried a higher risk of the disease.

A vitamin D_3 deficiency may be a reason for seasonal variations in mood, according to an article published in *Psychopharmacology.* The study involved forty-four student volunteers—thirty-four women and ten men between the ages of eighteen and forty-three—with a mean age of twenty-two.[31]

The research team gave the volunteers vitamin D_3 supplements at 0 IU, 400 IU, or 800 IU/day for five days during late winter in a double-blind study.

The central nervous system is a target organ for vitamin D, according to an article in *Schizophrenia Research.* The article suggests that low maternal vitamin D intake may adversely affect the developing fetal brain, leaving the offspring affected with schizophrenia, which is a psychotic disorder characterized by a loss of contact with the environment.[32]

To support this theory, the author reported an excess of schizophrenia during the winter months, when vitamin D levels are notoriously low; increased rates of the mental disorder in dark-skinned migrants to cold climates; and an increased rate of schizophrenia births in urban as opposed to rural areas, as well as an association between prenatal famine and schizophrenia, the author added.

Researchers have reported a lower mean 25(OH)D concentration in African American women than in white women, aged twenty to forty, according to Shanna Nesby-O'Dell and colleagues from the Centers for Disease Control and Prevention in Atlanta at various facilities. However, African American women have higher levels of bone density, fewer hip fractures, and longer delays in bone loss after menopause than do white women. Nevertheless, H. M. Perry and colleagues have observed that serum 25(OH)D was an independent predictor of femoral bone density in African American women.[33, 34]

Vitamin D Deficiency Is Now a Worldwide Pandemic

A pandemic is described as occurring over a wide geographic area and affecting an exceptionally high proportion of the population, such as the 1918–1919 influenza pandemic that killed an estimated 30 million people.

A vitamin D deficiency is now recognized as a worldwide pandemic, according to Michael F. Holick, MD, and Tai G. Chen of the Boston University Medical Center.*

This deficiency stems from a lack of appreciation that sun exposure in moderate amounts is the major source of vitamin D for most people, the authors added. In addition, foods that are fortified with vitamin D often have inadequate amounts of the vitamin to satisfy either a child's or an adult's vitamin D requirement.

Ongoing research suggests that children and adults should get at least 800–1,000 IU/day of vitamin D from dietary and supplementary sources when sunlight is unable to provide that amount, Holick and Chen said.

Major food sources of the vitamin are oily fish, such as salmon, mackerel, and herring; and fish oils, such as cod-liver oil. However, their recent study found that wild-caught salmon had, on average, 500–1,000 IU of vitamin D in 100 grams—3.5 ounces, or a typical serving—while farmed salmon contained only about 100–250 IU per serving.

The sunshine vitamin is poised to become the nutrient of the decade, if a host of recent findings are to be believed, according to Jane E. Brody in the *New York Times.***

Brody added that vitamin D, an essential nutrient found in a limited number of foods, has long been recognized for its role in creating strong bones, which is why it is added to milk. "Now a growing legion of medical researchers have raised strong doubts about the adequacy of current recommended levels of intake, from birth through the sunset years," she added.

Living in a warm climate doesn't necessarily ensure that you will get enough vitamin D, according to Elizabeth T. Jacobs of the Arizona Cancer Center in Tucson and colleagues at other facilities.*** "In spite of living in a region with a high chronic sun exposure, adults in southern Arizona are commonly deficient in vitamin D, especially dark-skinned people such as African-Americans and Hispanics," the researchers said.

Although a classic vitamin D deficiency leads to rickets and osteomalacia, and is uncommon in this population, recent research has associated suboptimal concentrations of circulating 25(OH)D with cancer, diabetes, and heart disease, the researchers added.

---

*Michael F. Holick, MD, and Tai C. Chen, "Vitamin D Deficiency: A Worldwide Problem with Health Consequences," *American Journal of Clinical Nutrition* 87 (2008): 1080S–1085S.

**Jane E. Brody, "An Oldie Vies for Nutrient of the Decade," *New York Times* (February 19, 2008): F7.

***Elizabeth T. Jacobs et al., "Vitamin D Insufficiency in Southern Arizona," *American Journal of Clinical Nutrition* 87 (2008): 608–613.

Concerning newborns, their 25(OH)D concentration is about one-half that of the mother's vitamin D. A risk factor for poor vitamin D status in early infancy is maternal vitamin D deficiency during pregnancy, which results in inadequate maternal transfer of vitamin D to the fetus and low infant stores.

In the study, the researchers evaluated 1,546 African American women and 1,426 white women, ages fifteen to forty-nine, who were not pregnant and who participated in the Third National and Nutrition Examination Survey (1988–1994). Low vitamin D status was defined as a serum 25-hydroxyvitamin D concentration less than 37.5 nmol/l.

It was found that hypovitaminosis D was around 42.4 percent among African American women and about 4.2 percent in the white women. Among the black women, low vitamin D levels were independently associated with consumption of milk or breakfast cereals—less than three times a week—no use of vitamin D supplements, season, urban residence, low body mass index, and no use of oral contraceptives. Even among the 243 African American volunteers who consumed an adequate intake of vitamin D from supplements—200 IU/day—almost 28.2 percent had hypovitaminosis D or low blood levels of the vitamin.

"The high prevalence of hypovitaminosis D among African American women warrants further examination of vitamin D recommendations for these women," the researchers said. "The determinants of hypovitaminosis D among women should be considered when these women are advised on dietary intake and supplement use."

In surveying 152 patients with gastrointestinal problems and 104 others with chronic liver disease, a mild deficiency was common and a severe deficiency—as defined by blood levels of 25-hydroxyvitamin D of more than 8 nmol/l—was seen in every disease category, according to the *Quarterly Journal of Medicine*.[35]

In those with Crohn's disease, deficiency was more prevalent than in those with inactive disease and in patients with chronic pancreatitis or pancreatic carcinoma, the researchers said. It was also reported that deficiency was more common in those with Crohn's disease who had been treated surgically than in those who had not had surgery.

In addition, patients with chronic liver disease, those with primary biliary cirrhosis, had lower blood levels of 25-hydroxyvitamin D than in those with Stage 1 and Stage 2 disease who had normal levels. Researchers also found that vitamin D levels were lower in those bothered by itching and jaundice.

Lesson No. 2

Current federal recommendations for adults, aged fifty-one to seventy, still call for the 400/IU day used in these studies. Yet research now shows that 700 to 1,000 IU/day of vitamin D appears necessary to reach the most healthy blood levels of the vitamin. A daily intake of 400 IU is now considered inadequate to prevent fractures, Collins continued.

Lesson No. 3

By the end of the trial, only 59 percent of the women were still taking their supplements as instructed. The women who actually took their calcium and vitamin D supplements had 29 percent fewer hip fractures.

Lesson No. 4

While no significant difference was seen in cancer risk, tumor characteristics, or reports of polyps in this study, a seven-year study is not enough time to see the effects on a disease that typically develops over ten to twenty years. However, it should be noted that the women who started the study with low blood levels of vitamin D developed more than twice as much colorectal cancer as those with the highest blood levels, Collins continued.

This evidence supports the idea that long-term vitamin D status may affect the risk for this cancer. The women with the lowest blood levels of vitamin D also tended to show the most benefit from supplements. Bottom line: longer duration of use and higher doses than now recommended might have produced truly significant effects in the women who lacked vitamin D.

Lesson No. 5

For bone health and lower colon cancer risk, meeting current recommendations for calcium and vitamin D is a good start, Collins said. For optimal wellness protection, add regular exercise, weight control, limited sodium intake, and a balanced diet, especially with plenty of fruits, vegetables, and whole grains daily.

Adequate intake of certain nutrients that are essential for bone metabolism—such as calcium and vitamin D—plays an important role in maintaining bone mass, according to Yannis Manios of Harokopio University in Athens, Greece, and colleagues at the University of Athens. With increasing age, however, both dietary calcium intake and intestinal calcium absorption decrease, and in the elderly, blood levels of vitamin D decline, mostly because of decreased sunlight exposure, which leads to a limited capacity for cutaneous vitamin D synthesis.[2]

"Combined with low dietary intake of vitamin D from foods, especially in countries without a mandatory fortification policy, these factors contribute to lower concentrations of vitamin D and, consequently, to accelerated bone loss and greater risk of bone fracture," the researchers said.

An abundance of clinical trials has indicated the beneficial effects of supplementation with calcium, vitamin D, or both, on the prevention of bone loss and on bone remodeling, but few studies have examined the effect of increases in the intakes of these nutrients through fortified foods and, especially, through dairy products, the research team continued.

In their study, 101 postmenopausal women were randomly assigned to a dairy intervention group (39), who were given each day 1,200 mg of calcium and 7.5 mcg of vitamin D_3 via fortified dairy products; a calcium supplement group (26), who received a total of 1,200 mg/day of calcium; and a control group (36).

The researchers reported that increases observed in blood concentrations of insulinlike growth factor I were greater in the dairy intervention group than in the two other groups, especially during the first five months of intervention. The decreases and increases observed during five and twelve months, respectively, in serum 25-hydroxyvitamin D were significant in all groups. Serum parathyroid hormone increased only in the controls. The parathyroid hormone, secreted by the parathyroid gland, is necessary for the regulation of calcium levels in the blood. The dairy intervention group had greater improvements in pelvis, total spine, and total body bone mineral density than did the other two groups.

"The application of a holistic intervention approach combining nutrition education and consumption of fortified dairy products for twelve months can induce more favorable changes in biochemical indexes of bone metabolism and bone mineral density than can calcium supplementation alone," the researchers added.

To investigate the relative importance of high calcium intake and serum 25-hydroxyvitamin D for calcium homeostasis, as determined by serum intact parathyroid hormone, Laufey Steingrimsdottir, PhD, at the University of Iceland in Reykjavik and colleagues at the Landspitali University Hospital in the same city, conducted a cross-sectional study of 2,310 Icelandic adults, who were divided into three age groups—thirty to forty-five; fifty to sixty-five; and seventy to eighty-five—who were recruited from February 2001 to January 2003. Each was given a food questionnaire that assessed the two nutrients and how frequently they were consumed.[3]

The participants were further divided into groups according to calcium intakes—less than 800 mg/day; 800–1,200 mg/day; and over 1,200 mg/day—and serum 25-hydroxyvitamin D levels of less than 10 ng/ml; 10 to 18 ng/ml; and over 18 ng/ml.

In all, 944 people completed all parts of the study. After adjusting for variables, parathyroid hormone was lowest in the group with the serum 25-hydroxyvitamin D level of more than 18 ng/ml, but highest in the group with a serum 25-hydroxyvitamin D level of less than 10 ng/ml.

"At the low blood 25-hydroxyvitamin D level—less than 10 ng/ml—calcium intake of less than 800 mg/day versus more than 1,200 mg/day—was significantly associated with higher serum parathyroid hormone levels, and at a calcium intake of more than 1,200 mg/day, there was a significant difference between the lowest and highest vitamin D groups," the researchers said.

The researchers added that as long as vitamin D status is ensured, calcium intake levels of more than 800 mg/day may be unnecessary for maintaining calcium metabolism. However, vitamin D supplements are necessary for adequate vitamin D levels, especially in northern climates.

Writing in the *New England Journal of Medicine,* Robert D. Utiger, MD, reported that vitamin D helps maintain calcium absorption and skeletal integrity and that the vitamin may be obtained from sunlight through the conversion of 7-dehydrocholesterol to previtamin D, which is then converted to vitamin D. Also, vitamin D from food sources or from the skin is converted to 25-hydroxyvitamin D in the liver and 1,25-dehydroxyvitamin D—the active hormone—in the kidneys.[4]

He went on to say that the serum half-life of 25-hydroxyvitamin D is longer than that of 1,25-dihydroxyvitamin D, in that it provides a better assessment of vitamin D intake and storage. Blood levels of 25-hydroxyvitamin D decrease with age, but go up slightly with sunlight exposure and vitamin D intake from foods and supplements.

He said that in the Framingham Study, 14 percent of the women and 6 percent of the men had low serum 25-hydroxyvitamin D stores. As an example, in 290 people with a mean age of sixty-two, poor vitamin D intake and remaining indoors contributed to low 25-hydroxyvitamin D amounts in the blood. Utiger found that 66 percent of those with low 25-hydroxyvitamin D amounts had estimated vitamin D intakes that were less than adequate for that age group.

A vitamin D deficiency is related to increased parathyroid hormone secretion, increased bone turnover, osteoporosis, and mild osteomalacia, he continued. Adults probably require 800 to 1,000 IU/day of the vitamin, which can be given as a single capsule of 5,000 IU or at a dose of 100,000 IU every four to six months. He suggested that the amount of vitamin D in supplemental multivitamins or calcium supplements should be increased substantially and that all adults should be advised to take supplements.

In an article in the *American Journal of Clinical Nutrition,* Mariana Cifuentes of Rutgers University, New Brunswick, New Jersey, and colleagues at St. Peters University Hospital in the same city evaluated the effect of six weeks of weight loss at two different amounts of calcium intake—1,000 mg/day and 1,800 mg/day—on calcium absorption, bone turnover, and bone-regulating hormones in overweight postmenopausal women.[5]

They reported that weight loss is associated with elevated calcium requirements, which, if met, could activate the calcium-parathyroid hormone axis to absorb more of the mineral. Normal intakes of the mineral during energy restriction result in inadequate total calcium absorption, and this could ultimately compromise calcium balance and bone mass, they said.

The relative increase in serum $1,25(OH)_2D$ with weight loss is intriguing, they added. Their measurements were done at an early stage of weight loss, and there could be an acute release of vitamin D stored in adipose tissue available for conversion to the active metabolite, they continued.

"Although vitamin D status was within normal range in our overweight subjects, it was shown that the obese have lower serum vitamin D concentrations and secondary hyperparathyroidism, possibly because of the deposit of vitamin D in adipose tissue," they noted. "In addition, we have shown higher $25(OH)D$ concentrations after energy restriction in obese but not in lean laboratory animals. Hence, increased serum vitamin D during weight loss could be expected."

As discussed in the *Journal of the American Geriatrics Society,* thirty-two African Americans, sixty-eight to ninety-three years of age, were evaluated for 25-hydroxyvitamin D levels, parathyroid hormones, osteocalcin, and calcitonin. They were compared with forty-three white Americans, who were seventy to eighty-nine years of age.[6]

The study found 25-hypervitaminosis D (excessive amounts) with secondary hyperthyroidism frequently occurred in the elderly African Americans. Osteocalcin, a measure of osteoblast activity, correlated with 25-hydroxyvitamin D and parathyroid hormone.

For osteocalcin, a protein found in bone and dentin, blood levels were lower in the African Americans than in the Caucasians, but serum calcium corrected for albumin and was higher in the blacks than in the whites.

The finding of lower calcitonin levels in the African Americans may put this group at higher risk of bone loss, explained Horace M. Perry III and colleagues at St. Louis University and Medical School in Missouri.

Perry added that there seem to be several differences in bone metabolism between Caucasians and African Americans. Therefore, vitamin D supplementation may be appropriate for older African Americans, as has been suggested for older Caucasians.

According to I. R. Reid, calcium supplements produce beneficial effects on bone mass among women throughout postmenopausal life, and they may reduce fracture rates by as much as 50 percent. Some of the most substantial reductions in fracture rate have been due to calcium and vitamin D supplements.[7]

In some studies, Reid added, 1,200 mg of calcium plus 800 IU/day of vitamin D have proved useful. In other studies, 500 mg/day of calcium and 700 IU/day of vitamin D have been recommended. Vitamin D status can be normalized in the frail elderly by encouraging them to walk outdoors for fifteen to thirty minutes in the sunlight, Reid said.

For the first five years following menopause, women lose bone rapidly, according to Bess Dawson-Hughes, MD, in the *Journal of Nutrition*. While high-dose calcium supplementation can modestly reduce cortical bone loss from long bones, this has little effect on the spine, she said.[8]

Vitamin D seems to enhance the effectiveness of supplemented calcium and the mineral usually benefits postmenopausal women who have the lowest dietary intake of the mineral and who are late coming to menopause, she added. However, in calcium-replete women, supplementation with vitamin D reduces bone loss and fracture incidence. In postmenopausal women, 1,000–1,500 mg/day of calcium and 400–800 IU/day of vitamin D can reduce bone loss, she continued.

Two of the most important nutrients for bone health are calcium and vitamin D; however, for women sixty-five and over, the RDA for calcium is 800 mg/day and for vitamin D, 200 IU/day, reported H. Karimi Kinyamu and colleagues at Creighton University School of Medicine in Omaha, Nebraska.[9]

"According to many nutritional surveys, a high proportion of the elderly in North America consume less than the RDA for both nutrients," the researchers said. "In addition, although calcium intake may be normal, calcium absorption is less efficient in the elderly, thereby limiting the amount of the mineral absorbed from the diet. Seniors are also at risk of vitamin D deficiency because of insufficient dietary intake, inadequate sun exposure, and impaired kidney synthesis of calcium."

In their study, the effect of dietary calcium and vitamin D on serum parathyroid hormone and vitamin D metabolism was evaluated in 376 women, ranging in age from sixty-five to seventy-seven. Their calcium intake was similar to the RDA amount of 800 mg/day. The mean vitamin D intake in 245 women not taking a vitamin D supplement was 141 IU/day, well below the RDA of 200 IU/day.

To test their hypothesis that vitamin D is more important than calcium in reducing serum parathyroid hormone, the source of dietary calcium intake was subdivided into milk, which is fortified with vitamin D, and nonmilk sources.

It was found that serum parathyroid hormone concentration was inversely correlated with calcium intake derived from milk, but not from nonmilk sources of calcium. Serum calcidiol correlated with milk calcium intake, but not with nonmilk calcium intake. Calcidiol is 25-hydroxycholecalciferol or calcifediol.

"Our study showed that milk is an important nutritional source of vitamin D in the elderly, providing almost 50 percent of the dietary vitamin D intake," the researchers continued. "An increase in vitamin D intake, either by an increase in milk intake or from vitamin D supplements, should increase serum calcidiol and decrease blood levels of parathyroid hormone."

They added that the results of their study suggest that no adequate intake of vitamin D played a more significant role than did the calcium intake (100–1,700 mg/day) in suppressing secondary hyperparathyroidism within the calcium intake range. Elderly women probably need to consume more than the current RDA of vitamin D (200 IU/day) to increase serum calcidiol and decrease serum parathyroid hormone to normal concentrations.

Unfortunately, many studies do not mention that, if the bones are not getting sufficient amounts of calcium from diet and supplements, the body simply leaches the mineral from the bones, thereby putting the patient at risk for fractures.

3.

Vitamin D and Women's Health

Concerns about vitamin D have resurfaced in medical and scientific literature because the prevalence of a vitamin D deficiency in the United States, especially among darkly pigmented people, has increased, explained Bruce W. Hollis and Carol L. Wagner of the Medical University of South Carolina in Charleston. The purpose of their review, as reported in the *American Journal of Clinical Nutrition,* was to focus on women during pregnancy and lactation.[1]

"The approximate dose of vitamin D during pregnancy and lactation is unknown, although it appears to be greater than the current reference intake of 200 to 400 IU/day," they said. "Doses less than 10,000 IU/day (250 mcg/day) for up to five months do not elevate circulating 25-hydroxyvitamin D to concentrations over 90 ng/ml, whereas doses less than 1,000 IU/day, in many cases, are inadequate for maintaining normal circulating 25-hydroxyvitamin D levels between 15 and 80 ng/ml."

They added that vitamin D plays no etiologic role in cardiac valvular disease, such as that observed in Williams syndrome, and, as such, animal models involving vitamin D intoxication that show an effect on cardiac disease are flawed and offer no insight into normal human physiology. Williams syndrome is a congenital disorder involving mental deficiency, mild growth deficiency, elevated blood calcium, hypersensitivity to vitamin D, and excess ingestion of the vitamin during pregnancy.

"In fact," they continued, "higher doses of vitamin D are necessary for a large segment of Americans to achieve concentrations equivalent to those in people who live and work in sun-rich environments."

From the available evidence, it is clear that the antirachitic (preventing rickets) activity of human milk is variable and it is affected by the season, maternal vitamin D intake, and race, they added. How, then, is the nutritional vitamin D status of neonates and infants affected if they are exclusively breastfed?

The researchers went on to say that at least one study (Cancela, et al.)[2] reported that circulating vitamin D levels in breastfed infants are directly related to the vitamin D content of the mother's milk. Available evidence suggests that if the vitamin D status of the lactating mother is adequate, her breastfeeding infant will maintain a "minimally normal" nutritional vitamin D status.

"The best example of this was given by Greer and Marshall,[3] who reported that white infants who were exclusively breastfed during the winter in a northern climate maintained a 'minimally normal' vitamin D status for six months," the researchers said. "However, circulating vitamin D actually decreased as their study continued and this decrease occurred in spite of a maternal vitamin D intake of around 700 IU/day."

In contrast, the South Carolina researchers continued, a Finnish study showed that maternal supplementation with 1,000 IU/day of vitamin D resulted in a minimal increase in circulating vitamin D in breastfeeding infants. These same researchers repeated a similar study with 2,000 IU/day and found that the vitamin D status of the breastfeeding infants improved significantly.

"Our group recently performed similar studies, supplementing lactating women with 2,000 or 4,000 IU/day of vitamin D for three months," Hollis and Wagner added. "We found that high dose maternal vitamin D supplementation not only improved the nutritional vitamin D status of breastfeeding infants, but also elevates the maternal concentrations into the mid-normal range. It is noteworthy that, in the Finnish study, the authors added a disclaimer that 2,000 IU/day is far higher than the RDA for lactating mothers and so its safety over prolonged periods is not known and should be examined in further studies."

While this concern was valid when the Finnish study was published in 1986, findings by Reinhold Vieth and colleagues[4] and Robert P. Heaney and colleagues[5] have shown that vitamin D intakes of less than 10,000 IU/day are safe for prolonged periods—up to five months.

Hollis and Wagner concluded that "We believe that it is time to reexamine the understated dietary reference intake (DRI) of vitamin D for lactating mothers."

Recent studies have suggested that vitamin D may have value in preventing and treating cancer and autoimmune diseases, reported Carlos A. Camargo Jr. of Massachusetts General Hospital and Harvard Medical School in Boston and colleagues at other facilities. It has also been shown, especially in the northeastern United States, that a large proportion of Americans have an inadequate vitamin D intake. Another public health problem in the region is asthma; the Northeast region has the highest rates in the nation. Nationally, the prevalence of asthma has increased from about 3 percent in the 1970s to around 8 percent in recent years.[6]

The research team theorized that a higher maternal intake of vitamin D during pregnancy is associated with a lower risk of recurrent wheezing in children at three years of age. To investigate this hypothesis, they recruited 1,194 mother-child pairs in Project Viva—a prospective prebirth cohort study in Massachusetts. Vitamin D intake was ascertained through a food frequency questionnaire. The primary outcome was a recurrent wheeze; that is, a positive asthma predictive index or more than two wheezing attacks among children with a personal diagnosis of eczema or a parental history of asthma.

The mean total vitamin D intake during pregnancy was around 548 IU/day, plus or minus 167 IU/day. By age three, 186 children (16 percent) in the study had a recurrent wheeze. When compared with mothers in the lowest quartile of daily intake (median 356 IU), those in the highest quartile (724 IU) had a lower risk of having a child with a recurrent wheeze.

The researchers also found that an increase of 100 IU of vitamin D intake was associated with a lower risk, regardless of whether the vitamin came from diet or supplements.

"We hypothesized that higher vitamin D intakes are protective against asthmas in populations with inadequate vitamin D intake," the researchers continued. "In addition to the regional similarities, vitamin D insufficiency is more common among African Americans and among the obese. Temporal trends in the adoption of sunscreen use and in reductions in milk intake also support the hypothesized link between vitamin D and asthma."

The onset of asthma occurred before age six in 80–90 percent of the cases and before the age of three in 70 percent of the patients, the research team added. While the connection between vitamin D and asthma remains elusive, the role of maternal diet on risk of the disease in a mother's offspring is a particularly intriguing topic for research, given the growing evidence on the developmental origins of health and disease and the early age of asthma onset.

"Pregnant and lactating women are known to be at higher risk of vitamin D deficiency and our findings provide additional support for efforts to improve the nutritional status of this population, including recommended intakes of over

400 IU/day," the researchers said. "The low cost and safety of vitamin D containing foods and supplements could provide a very attractive intervention for the primary prevention of asthma."

Women who take vitamin D and calcium supplements seem to lower their risk of stress fractures, according to the February 20, 2007 issue of the *New York Times*.[7]

A research team, headed by Joan Lappe, MD, followed the health of more than five thousand female Navy recruits, who were participating in eight weeks of basic training. One group received 2,000 mg/day of calcium and 800 IU/day of vitamin D, while the others were given look-alike pills.

The study, presented at a meeting of the Orthopaedic Research Society, reported that the women who took the supplements were about 25 percent less likely to have a stress fracture when compared with the controls. If these findings were applied to all 14,000 women who passed through the training camp over two years, this would have prevented 130 fractures. The study also suggested that the recruits who reported a history of performing weight-bearing exercises were less likely to have a fracture.

There is mounting evidence that, in the absence of adequate exposure to sunlight—over 1,000 IU/day—dietary or supplemental vitamin D is required in adults to prevent vitamin D deficiency, according to Hussein F. Saadi of United Arab Emirates University in Al Aim and colleagues in Cincinnati. However, they added, a critical factor affecting the outcome is strict adherence to medications.[8]

"Our clinical experience indicates a low compliance with vitamin D supplement use in women in the United Arab Emirates (UAE)," the researchers said. "In a survey of prenatal multivitamin supplement use, only 40 percent of the Middle Eastern women, who delivered at term in a maternity hospital, reported using their prescribed prenatal vitamins in the last trimester of their pregnancy."

They added that intermittent high-dose regimens could overcome low compliance and that a dose of 50,000 IU/day of vitamin D_2 has been suggested as effective in maintaining acceptable vitamin D status. Since the biological half-life of 25(OH)D is effectively one to two months, dosing less than once every two months may generate large fluctuations in 25(OH)D concentrations that may not be desirable or effective.

The object of their study was to determine the effectiveness and safety of two vitamin D supplementation regimens—a daily dose of 2,000 IU or a monthly oral dose of 60,000 IU of vitamin D_2—in improving the vitamin D status of a convenience sample of lactating and nulliparous (nonpregnant) women residing in the UAE.

The study involved healthy lactating (ninety) and nulliparous (eighty-eight) women, who were randomly assigned to receive either 2,000 IU/day of vitamin D_2 or 60,000 IU in one dose for three months. At the beginning of the study, most of the women had a vitamin D deficiency—less than 50 nmol/l—and the supplementation increased blood levels of the vitamin over 50 nmol/l in twenty-one (30 percent) of seventy-one women at the conclusion of the study. While there is abundant sunshine in the region, women tend to wear traditional clothing that inhibits the conversion of vitamin D from the sun.

"Vitamin D_2 supplementation in our study increased blood levels of the vitamin significantly; however, these concentrations became acceptable—over 50 nmol/l—in only a small proportion of the women studied," the researchers continued. "In the absence of adequate sunlight exposure and if the more potent vitamin D_3 preparation is not available, higher doses of vitamin D_2 than currently studied may be needed. Monthly dosing appears to be a safe and effective alternative to daily dosing, especially in those from whom poor compliance is anticipated."

Writing in the *American Journal of Clinical Nutrition* in 2007, Puneet Arora of Queen's Park Hospital, Blackburn, United Kingdom, and Ramandeep S. Arora of the Royal Manchester Children's Hospital in the same country, referred to a previous article in the journal concerning pregnant non-Western women in the Netherlands and vitamin D deficiency (I. M. van der Meer, et al.).[9, 10] The Aroras were concerned about the conflicting recommendations from the Department of Health and the National Institute of Clinical Excellence in the United Kingdom and antenatal vitamin D supplementation.

"Several studies have shown the benefit of vitamin D supplementation in pregnant women in the United Kingdom, including a double-blind randomized, controlled trial that showed increases in maternal serum 25-hydroxycholecalciferol concentrations following vitamin D supplementation," they said. "Maternal nutritional status also benefitted as assessed by maternal weight gain and concentrations of vitamin A binding protein and thyroid binding prealbumin."

They added that cord blood 25-hydroxycholecalciferol concentrations also improved. Following birth, there was a significantly lower incidence of hypocalcemia—low blood levels of calcium—in the supplemented group and evidence of significant improvement in weight and length of the infant up to one year of age.

Considering the evidence, they continued, pregnant British Asian women should be routinely supplemented with vitamin D, and the Department of Health (DOH) recommends, based on the Committee on Medical Aspects of Food (COMA) Policy, that all pregnant and breastfeeding women should receive 400 IU/day of vitamin D.

Unfortunately, the National Institute of Clinical Evidence (NICE) has recommended, based on a Cochrane Database System Review, that there is insufficient evidence to evaluate the effectiveness of vitamin D in pregnancy and, in the absence of evidence of benefit, vitamin D supplementation should not be offered routinely to pregnant women.

"The same Cochrane review, however, recommends that vitamin D supplementation in the later part of pregnancy should be considered in vulnerable groups, such as Asian women living in Northern Europe and, possibly, those living in geographic areas with long winters, such as the United Kingdom and the Netherlands," the Aroras continued.

They went on to say that the contradictory statements from DOH and NICE have led to confusion in antenatal clinics in hospitals and in general practice. In a recent survey of general practice in the Thames Valley area and Lambeth— where 67.9 percent of medical practices had Asian and African Caribbean populations comprising over 8 percent of the population—none were supplementing pregnant women with vitamin D.

They concluded, based on the evidence, that all pregnant and breastfeeding women should be given 400 IU/day of vitamin D.

As reported in the *International Federation of Gynecology and OBS,* 666 pregnant women were given calcium at an elemental dose of 156 or 312 mg/day and vitamin D at 0.5 mcg three times daily by mouth. Those given the supplements had an incidence of preeclampsia of 10.9 percent, compared with the controls of 16.9 percent. Preeclampsia is a serious condition in which high blood pressure, fluid retention, and protein in the urine develop in the second half of a pregnancy. The authors concluded that both the vitamin D and the calcium therapy were successful in preventing preeclampsia for women at high risk.[11]

At the Medical College of Wisconsin in Milwaukee, Dwight P. Cruikshank, MD, and colleagues, evaluated fifteen women with preeclampsia who were treated with magnesium sulfate during labor, as well as the relationship of calcium, vitamin D, and parathyroid hormone status.[12]

The women were given a loading dose of magnesium of 4–6 g over thirty minutes, followed by a maintenance dose of 1–3 g/hour. All the patients were on the mineral for at least twelve hours before delivery.

The magnesium infusions resulted in reducing both maternal and fetal calcium levels, and both mother and fetus responded with increased 1,25-dihydroxyvitamin D and parathyroid hormone levels, which may, in turn, prevent fetal and secondary hypocalcemia.

The researchers concluded that maternal hypomagnesemia causes relative maternal hypocalcemia, which is balanced by an increased maternal 1,25-dihydroxycalciferol (vitamin D_3) and parathyroid hormone levels.

African American women living in northern latitudes apparently don't manufacture enough vitamin D during the summer to carry them through winter months, and they need to increase their vitamin D intake, according to a study by Susan Harris and colleagues at the Jean Mayer USDA Human Nutrition Research Center on Aging, Tufts University in Boston.[13]

The researchers reported that African American women had about half as much 25-hydroxyvitamin D circulating in their blood during the year as white women. In evaluating fifty-one African American women and thirty-nine white women living in the Boston area, the researchers noted that, in winter, when vitamin D levels are notoriously low, parathyroid hormone was raised only in the African American women. The hormone signals when blood calcium is low, and it can stimulate loss of the mineral from the bones.

Vitamin D supplementation may be of benefit in preventing osteoporosis in postmenopausal black women, according to the *Journal of Clinical Endocrinology and Metabolism.* The study involved ten healthy postmenopausal black women, who were given 20 mcg/day of vitamin D_3 for three months.[14]

At the end of the study, mean blood levels of 25-hydroxyvitamin D had increased from 24 to 63 nmol/l. The vitamin raised 25-hydroxyvitamin D levels and reduced secondary hyperparathyroidism and bone turnover.

In an article in the *Journal of the American Medical Association,* ninety-eight postmenopausal women were admitted for hip replacement; thirty had acute hip fractures, and sixty-eight were having elective joint replacement at Brigham and Women's Hospital in Boston. Seventeen of the joint replacement patients had osteoporosis and fifty-one did not.[15]

It was found that the women with hip fractures had lower levels of 25-hydroxyvitamin D than women with or without osteoporosis receiving joint replacement. It was also reported that parathyroid hormone levels were higher in the women with hip fractures. In addition, fifteen women with hip fractures had vitamin D levels that were deficient. N-telopeptide, a marker of bone resorption, was greater in the women with hip fractures, compared with elective nonosteoporotic controls.

Since the postmenopausal women with hip fractures showed occult (hidden) vitamin D deficiency, replacing vitamin D and suppressing parathyroid hormone, at the time of fracture, may help reduce future risk and enhance hip repair, according to Meryl S. LeBoff, MD, the *JAMA* study author.

As reported in the *New Zealand Medical Journal,* K. A. McAuley, MD, and colleagues, evaluated thirty-eight elderly patients over the age of seventy and found that hip density was correlated with 25-hydroxyvitamin D levels as the study began. In the summer, ten of the thirty-eight patients had vitamin D levels below the reference range for healthy adults. Six patients decided not to continue with the study.[16]

In the winter, twenty-two of the remaining thirty-two women had blood levels of the vitamin below the reference range. Those with low levels of vitamin D were given halibut oil tablets containing 400 IU/day of vitamin D_3 to improve their vitamin D levels.

The researchers reported that vitamin D supplements are inexpensive and effective and should be considered for those seventy and over who are at risk for hip fractures, especially those who live in temperate climates.

In an article in the *European Journal of Clinical Nutrition,* a research team evaluated 2,319 women between 1993 and 1997. It was found that daily calcium intake was 798 mg among heavy smokers—over twenty cigarettes a day—882 mg among moderate smokers—one to nineteen cigarettes a day—and 945 mg among those who never smoked.[17]

Of the heavy smokers, 21 percent did not eat yogurt, compared with 10 percent for never-smokers. Among yogurt eaters, heavy smokers consumed 90 mg/day of calcium from yogurt compared with 115 mg/day for those who never smoked. Smokers ate more butter and cream or milk than never-smokers; however, these foods were minor sources of the mineral.

Fish was the main source for higher intakes of vitamin D in never-smokers, compared with heavy and moderate smokers. Following five or more years of not smoking, with regard to calcium and vitamin D intake, intakes were 900 mg/day and 2.55 mcg/day, respectively. The researchers added that females who currently smoke have lower dietary intakes of calcium and vitamin D than never-smokers.

Researchers at Sri Venkateswara Institute of Medical Sciences in Tirupati, India, previously (C. V. Harinarayan et al., "Vitamin D Status in Primary Hyperthyroidism in India," *Clinical Endocrinology* 43 [1995]: 351–358) reported on the prevalence of low vitamin D concentrations in a group of healthy Indians and in patients with primary hyperthyroidism. It was surprising to find low concentrations of vitamin D in healthy people in a country with abundant sunshine.[18]

The current study involved 943 urban and 205 rural healthy people in Tirupati in Southern Andhra Pradesh, India, with a latitude of 13.4 degrees north and a longitude of 79.2 degrees east. The average duration of cloud-free sunshine is between eight and ten hours/day throughout the year, with the solar zenith angle at 9.92 degrees in summer and 38.2 degrees in the winter.

The research team found that dietary calcium intake of both the urban and rural populations was low compared with the recommended dietary allowances issued by the Indian Council of Medical Research. Dietary calcium and phosphorus were significantly lower in rural adults than in urban adults, and the dietary phytate-to-calcium ratio was higher in rural than in urban people.

The vitamin D levels of the rural subjects were higher than those in the urban subjects in both men and women. In the rural volunteers, vitamin D–deficient, insufficient, and sufficient levels were observed in 44, 39.5, and 16.5 percent of the men and 70, 29, and 1 percent of the women, respectively.

For the urban population, vitamin D–deficient, insufficient, and sufficient levels were reported in 62, 26, and 12 percent of the men and 75, 19, and 6 percent of the women, respectively.

"Low dietary calcium intake and vitamin D concentrations were associated with deleterious effects on bone mineral homeostatis," the researchers added. "Prospective longitudinal studies are required to assess the effect of bone mineral density, a surrogate marker for fracture risk and fracture rates."

It is interesting that Indians, along with other Asians and Africans, make chapattis, which consist mostly of whole wheat flour and water made into pancakes. These breads contain phytates, which unite with calcium and other minerals, causing them to be excreted unused.

As reported in *Headache,* Susan Thys-Jacobs, MD, of Mount Sinai Medical Center in New York, evaluated two women whose premenstrual syndrome (PMS) and migraine headaches improved with calcium and vitamin D. The first case involved a thirty-three-year-old woman who had frequent migraine headaches and PMS. The second patient was a forty-year-old woman with a history of migraines with aura and a ten-year history of PMS.[19]

The first patient was given a combination of 1,600 IU/day of cholecalciferol (vitamin D_3) and 1,200 mg/day of calcium because of low vitamin D levels. Within two months, the migraine headache attacks were significantly improved, along with her PMS symptoms.

A repeat of her 25-hydroxyvitamin D level showed a significant increase into the low-normal range of 17.3 ng/ml. Treatment with a higher oral dose of vitamin D_2 at 50,000 IU/week resulted in the elimination of her PMS symptoms.

In the second patient, vitamin D and calcium levels were normal, but she was placed on 1,200 IU/day of vitamin D and 1,200 mg/day of calcium for three months. There was a significant reduction in her migraine headaches as well as her PMS symptoms. Her 25-hydroxyvitamin D level increased with the supplementation and further migraine attacks were headed off immediately when chewing the equivalent of 1,200 and 1,600 mg of elemental calcium, Dr. Thys-Jacobs said.

4.

Vitamin D and Children's Health

Poor vitamin D status has recently been linked to diseases such as breast, colorectal, ovarian, and prostate cancers; cardiovascular disease; multiple sclerosis; diabetes; and the metabolic syndrome; as well as to increased falls and impaired neuromuscular function. These findings have important implications, since vitamin D insufficiency has been estimated to be present in 20–60 percent of adults over the age of fifty. However, little is known about vitamin D requirements for children, and what is known is primarily based on cross-sectional studies, reported Catherine M. Willis and colleagues at the University of Georgia at Athens in the *American Journal of Clinical Nutrition* in 2007.[1, 2]

The aim of their study was to determine blood levels of 25(OH)D in prepubertal black and white girls living in northeast Georgia, to determine whether vitamin D concentrations change with increasing age.

Blood levels of vitamin D were collected from girls ranging in age from four to eight who participated in a University of Georgia Childhood Bone Study in Athens, which is located at latitude 34 degrees north. The volunteers had no serious health problems and they did not use medications known to alter bone metabolism. The girls represented all racial groups.

It was found that plasma 25(OH)D levels—less than 80 nmol/l—were observed in 75 percent of the girls; however, blood levels of the vitamin decreased with increasing age, independent of race, the researchers said. Blood levels of the vitamin were higher in whites than in blacks, and the amount of the difference depended on the season. The effects of age, race, and season on vitamin D levels remained significant when dietary calcium, vitamin D, and physical activity were used as covariates after adjustment for fat-free soft tissue (FFST). Whether FFST requires additional vitamin D during growth remains to be determined.

"Circulating concentrations of 25(OH)D declined with growth and this may be related to the increased utilization of vitamin D by soft tissue," the researchers added. "In this sample of young females living in the southeastern United States, 18 percent had blood levels of vitamin D that fell below 50 nmol/l at least once during the study. Further investigation into the utilization of 1,25-dihydroxyvitamin D by muscle and the subsequent effect on circulating vitamin D concentrations in children may help to elucidate the relation between FFST mass and vitamin D status."

Ninety-one healthy eight-year-old Caucasian girls were enrolled in the vitamin D supplemented group and fifteen acted as controls, reported the *Journal of Clinical Endocrinology and Metabolism.* The researchers found that the vitamin D supplemented girls had higher bone mineral density at the level of radial metaphysis (a conical section of bone), femoral neck, and femoral trochanter.[3]

At the lumbar spine level, these measurements were similar between the two groups; however, in the supplemented group, femoral neck bone mineral density remained higher. Supplemental vitamin D in infancy was associated with increased bone mineral density at specific skeletal sites in prepubertal Caucasian girls. The supplemented group was given 400 IU/day of vitamin D as cholecalciferol for a median period of twelve months.

In an article in *Primary Care and Cancer,* researchers reported that many teenage girls do not get enough calcium and vitamin D. In animal studies, at least, it has been suggested that reduced levels of these nutrients during this high period of growth can increase the risk of breast cancer.[4]

It is theorized that, because the mammary gland matures during adolescence, a high intake of fats and low intakes of calcium and vitamin D could increase the risk of breast cancer.

According to the American Academy of Pediatrics, 200 IU/day of vitamin D is recommended for the following:[5]

1. All breastfed infants, unless they are weaned, should receive at least 500 ml/day of vitamin D–fortified formula or milk.

2. All nonbreastfed infants who are given less than 500 ml of vitamin D–fortified formula or milk.

3. Children and adolescents who are not getting regular sunlight exposure or who do not ingest at least 500 ml/day of vitamin D–fortified milk or who do not take supplements containing at least 200 IU/day of vitamin D.

It is well recognized that adequate stores of vitamin D are critical for musculoskeletal health and the best indicator of vitamin D stores is the serum concentration of calcidiol or 25-hydroxyvitamin D—25(OH)D—according to Francis L. Weng of the University of Pennsylvania School of Medicine in Philadelphia and colleagues at various facilities in the United States.[6, 7, 8]

"When circulating 25(OH)D concentrations are inadequate, a state known as hypovitaminosis D, intestinal calcium absorption and bone mineralization are impaired," Weng said. "More severe deficits in vitamin D lead to clinical myopathy, osteomalacia in adults, and rickets in children."

The objective of the study by Weng and colleagues was to determine the prevalence of and factors associated with low concentrations of vitamin D in children and adolescents. Blood levels of 25(OH)D were measured in 382 healthy volunteers, six to twenty-one years of age, living in the northeastern United States.

It was found that median concentration of 25(OH)D was 28 ng/ml, and 55 percent of the volunteers had vitamin D concentrations of less than 30 ng/ml. The vitamin D concentrations were inversely correlated with parathyroid hormone concentrations, but were not significantly correlated with 1,25-dihydroxyvitamin D levels.

In this multivariable model, older age, black race, wintertime study visit, and total daily vitamin D intake—less than 200 IU/day—were associated with low vitamin D concentrations. Fat and lean body mass were not independently associated with vitamin D status in this healthy weight sample, the researchers added.

"Hypovitaminosis D remains an under-recognized problem in the general population and it is poorly defined in children," the researchers continued. "Recent studies showed inadequate circulating 25(OH)D concentrations in adult medical inpatients, postmenopausal women, and free-living adults. In the pediatric population, several studies have documented low blood levels of vitamin D in adolescents living in Boston, Cleveland, and Maine; in infants and toddlers; in Alaska; and in children of primary school age in Lebanon."

The researchers added that, of substantial concern, given the current obesity epidemic, is that obesity in children was also shown to be associated with decreased 25(OH)D concentrations.

Low serum 25(OH)D levels are prevalent in otherwise healthy children and adolescents in the mid-Atlantic United States and are related to low vitamin D intake, race, and season, the researchers concluded.

Over 330 children with developmental disabilities, who were or were not ambulatory and were or were not given anticonvulsants, were evaluated by Marion Taylor Baer and colleagues; their study was published in the *American Journal of Clinical Nutrition.* When compared with thirty-four normal control children, a high percentage of the children had intakes below the recommended dietary allowance for calcium (56 percent) and vitamin D (70 percent).[9]

Vitamin D intake was positively associated with serum calcium and calcidiol concentrations, and ambulatory status was a significant predictor of calcium and calcidiol status, the researchers said.

The research team added that all nonambulatory children may be at risk for low serum calcidiol and osteopenia; therefore, they should be routinely monitored with an eye toward vitamin D supplementation.

To meet vitamin D requirements, newborns who live in the northern latitudes are very dependent on body stores and dietary supplies, according to Francis Mimouni, MD, of Magee-Women's Hospital in Pittsburgh. Also, human milk contains significantly less vitamin D and calcifediol than fortified formulas, and vitamin D deficiency in rickets is almost exclusively reported in breastfed, mostly black infants. Calcifediol—25-hydroxycholecalciferol—is more potent than vitamin D_3, the researcher said.[10]

Although Mimouni supports a reduction in exposure of newborns to unprotected sunlight, this recommendation should be followed by administration of daily vitamin D supplements for breastfed infants, since the amount of endogenous synthesis with the use of sunblock is unknown.

Vitamin D deficiency leads to secondary hyperparathyroidism, which has a negative effect on bone metabolism in the elderly; however, the effect of serum 25-hydroxyvitamin D concentrations on parathyroid hormone concentrations and bone mineral density has not been well studied in adolescents, said Terhi A. Outila and colleagues at the University of Helsinki in Finland. High blood levels of vitamin D have been found in the summer and low concentrations in the winter in both young and old people, reflecting the amount of sun exposure they receive.[11]

In their study, the Finnish researchers evaluated the effect of vitamin D status on serum intact parathyroid hormone concentrations and bone metabolism in 178 healthy female adolescents, ranging in age from fourteen to sixteen.

The study was conducted in Helsinki—60 degrees north—during the winter. On the basis of the relation between serum 25(OH)D and parathyroid hormone concentrations, blood levels of vitamin D—over 40 nmol/l—were needed to keep parathyroid hormone levels low.

The research team reported that 110 girls (61.8 percent) had serum 25(OH)D concentrations less than 40 nmol/l, and 24 volunteers (13.5 percent) were considered vitamin D–deficient when the serum 25(OH)D concentration of 25 nmol/l was used as a cutoff. Those with serum 25(OH)D levels below 40 nmol/l had low mean forearm bone mineral density at both the radial and ulnar sites.

The researchers concluded that a large percentage of adolescent females have low vitamin D status during the winter in Finland, which seems to have a negative effect on their bone health.

Hyperparathyroidism is overactivity of the parathyroid glands, which produce parathyroid hormone. The hormone, along with vitamin D and calcitonin—a hormone produced by the thyroid gland—controls the level of calcium in the blood. Overproduction of parathyroid hormone elevates calcium in the blood by removing the mineral from bones, thereby resulting in osteoporosis and osteomalacia.[12]

Children and adolescents with Crohn's disease are at an increased risk of impaired bone mineralization, according to Timothy A. Santongo and colleagues of Children's Memorial Hospital, Northwestern University in Chicago and the Children's Hospital of Pennsylvania, University of Pennsylvania in Philadelphia. The peak incidence of Crohn's disease coincides with adolescence, which is a critical period of secretion of bone mass and skeletal maturation.[13]

In their study, the researchers examined the prevalence of and risk factors for low blood levels of vitamin D in children, adolescents, and young adults with Crohn's disease. Hypovitaminosis D was defined as a blood concentration of 25-hydroxyvitamin D (25(OH)D) less than 38 nmol/l.

There were 112 volunteers enrolled in the study, of whom 44 were females and 101 were white. There were 9 African American males and 2 others of other ethnicity. Hypovitaminosis D was detected in 18 subjects, including 56 percent of the African Americans and 13 percent of the whites. Of the participants, 35 were enrolled in the winter, 25 in the spring, 21 in the summer, and 31 in the fall. The girls were 5 to 22 years old.

Mean serum 25(OH)D concentrations tended to increase as the seasons progressed from winter to fall, and there was a higher prevalence of hypovitaminosis D in those with Crohn's disease involvement limited to the upper gastrointestinal tract, compared with those with other patterns of anatomical involvement, the researchers continued.

Low blood levels of vitamin D were associated with a greater lifetime exposure to glucocorticoid therapy. This is a steroid prescribed for its anti-inflammatory effect.

"Pure growth and nutritional status, delayed pubertal development, increased inflammatory cytokines, and glucocorticoid therapy all commonly occur in pediatric patients with Crohn's disease and negatively affect bone mineralization," the researchers added. "Furthermore, malabsorption of dietary vitamin D may occur in this disease and other inflammatory disorders that involve the small intestine."

The researchers went on to say that, to optimize nutritional care, serum 25(OH)D levels should be assessed in children, adolescents, and young adults with Crohn's disease, and vitamin D supplementation should be considered in those with low concentrations.

Commenting on the Santongo et al. study, John N. Udall Jr. of Louisiana State University and Children's Hospital in New Orleans, said that Crohn's disease early in life is associated with decreased blood levels of vitamin D. He added that among patients with Crohn's disease who have had portions of their small intestine resected, 60 percent have low blood levels of vitamin D. This contributes to osteoporosis and osteopenia.[14]

"Among those with inflammatory bowel disease, those with Crohn's disease are more likely to develop low bone mineral density than those with ulcerative colitis," Udall said. "The etiology involves malabsorption, steroid therapy, inflammatory mediators, hyperalimentation, and hypogonadism."

He added that the overall vitamin D status is best determined by the serum 25-hydroxyvitamin D concentration. Once adults with Crohn's disease have begun corticosteroid therapy, vitamin D_3 supplementation at 400 IU by mouth twice daily should be initiated, and this regimen should be considered for younger patients.

"When steroid therapy is begun, the risk of osteoporosis increases dramatically and the long term use of steroids is to be discouraged," he said. "Steroids should not be used for maintenance therapy."

Young adults with an HIV infection (pre-AIDs) are at an increased risk of osteopenia and osteoporosis; immune activation and antiretroviral therapy may underlie this phenomenon, reported Charles B. Stephensen of the University of California at Davis and colleagues at various locations. Changes in vitamin D metabolism due to HIV infection may also be a factor, since vitamin D is required for bone health maintenance and for adequate tissue function.[15]

"Vitamin D affects the development and function of cells of the immune system that help to control HIV infection, including macrophages and T-lymphocytes," Stephensen said.

The Reaching for Excellence in Adolescent Health (REACH) study examined many aspects of HIV infection in those fourteen to eighteen years of age, who were recruited in thirteen U.S. cities.

"Dietary quality in many REACH volunteers did not meet current recommendations, which raises questions about their vitamin D intake," the researchers continued. "This question is especially timely because recent studies suggest that vitamin D insufficiency in the U.S. is more widespread than was previously appreciated. Another reason for concern about the vitamin D status in our participants is that about three-fourths of the REACH volunteers are black, which in itself is a risk factor for the development of a vitamin D deficiency."

In the study, 74 percent were female and 72 percent were black. Mean vitamin D intake from food was 30 percent greater in HIV positive subjects than in the HIV negative people. The prevalence of vitamin D supplement use was 29 percent, and it did not differ significantly by HIV status. The prevalence of a vitamin D insufficiency—plasma 25(OH)D of less than 37.5 nmol/l—in the volunteers was 87 percent, that is, 312 out of 359 people.

"The prevalence of vitamin D insufficiency was alarmingly high in the adolescent and young adult members of the REACH cohort," the researchers concluded. "Low plasma 25(OH)D concentrations were associated with race, obesity, season—winter or spring—living in a northern city and low vitamin D intake."

Since vitamin D intake in the REACH subjects was similar to a nationally representative sample, it may be that limited sun exposure in a poor, urban environment is the factor that accounts for the higher than expected prevalence of vitamin D insufficiency in REACH subjects, the researchers added.

In evaluating thirty women one to four hours after giving birth, twenty-nine had low blood levels of vitamin D—less than 30 nmol/l—and thirteen had high serum parathyroid hormone levels, greater than 5.5 pmol/l. The median range of ionized calcium in the blood was 1.23 nmol/l, according to a study published in *Early Human Development*.[16]

The researchers reported a positive correlation between the level of ionized calcium in the maternal blood and the crown-to-heel length of the infant. They added that vitamin D deficiency, through an effect on maternal calcium homeostasis, may influence fetal growth.

At the Ulleval Hospital in Oslo, Norway, a $3\frac{1}{2}$-month-old infant was found to have a severe vitamin D deficiency, low blood levels of calcium, abnormally high levels of phosphorus in the blood, a dilated left ventricle, and congestive heart failure, reported *Acta Pediatrica*. The child also had a depressed thyroid function.[17]

The child was treated with calcium gluconate infusions, IV albumin, digoxin, and furosemide. Anticoagulant drugs were also prescribed, along with calcitriol (vitamin D_3) at 25 mcg/day for the first day in the hospital and then for three weeks afterward. Treatment was then continued with cholecalciferol (vitamin D_3) at 40 mcg/day for the following eight weeks.

The child improved dramatically. She was three years old at the time the article was written and receiving no medications. While myocardial function is normal, she does have some motor delay. The authors believe that her transitory congestive heart failure was caused by severe vitamin D deficiency, which produced low levels of calcium in the blood.

Chromatography was used to measure vitamin D in samples of thirteen brands of milk with various fat contents and five brands of infant formula purchased at local supermarkets, reported Michael F. Holick, PhD, MD, and colleagues at Boston University School of Medicine in Massachusetts.[18]

It was found that twelve of the forty-two samples of thirteen brands of milk, and none of the ten samples of the five brands of infant formula, contained from 80 percent to 120 percent of the amount of vitamin D shown on the label. In addition, twenty-six of the forty-two milk samples contained less than 80 percent of the amount claimed on the label. No vitamin D was found in three of fourteen samples of fat-free milk.

One milk sample, labeled as containing vitamin D_2 (ergocalciferol) actually contained vitamin D_3 (cholecalciferol). Seven of the ten samples of infant formula had more than 200 percent of the amount stated on the label. The sample with the highest concentrations of the vitamin contained 419 percent of the stated amount.

The authors concluded that milk and infant preparations rarely contain the amount of vitamin D stated on the label and, therefore, may be either underfortified or overfortified. They added that better monitoring of fortification is necessary, since both underfortification and overfortification may be hazardous to an infant's health.

In a study at the University of Jyvaskyla, Finland, Sulin Cheng and a research team from the United States and Finland evaluated the blood levels of vitamin D and parathyroid hormone with bone mineral content and bone mineral density at different sites, and the relation between 25(OH)D and parathyroid hormone in early pubertal and prepubertal Finnish girls.[19]

The 193 girls, ranging in age from ten to twelve, resided in Jyvaskyla, Finland, which is located at a latitude of 62 degrees north. It was found that 32 percent of the girls were vitamin D–deficient, and 46 percent of them had an insufficient blood concentration of the vitamin. The girls in the deficient groups also had significantly lower cortical volumetric bone mineral density of the distal radius and tibia shaft.

It was also reported that high parathyroid hormone concentrations were associated with low total body apparent mineral density and urinary calcium excretion.

"Using a cutoff of 25 nmol/l for serum 25(OH)D concentrations, we found that 32 percent of the girls, who had an average calcium intake of 733 mg/day, were deficient in vitamin D," the researchers added. "An additional 46 percent of the girls were considered to be vitamin D insufficient on the basis of 25(OH)D concentrations of 26 to 40 nmol/l."

The research team said they found that, in the present study, a substantial number of ten- to twelve-year-old girls from central Finland who had a low calcium intake were either deficient in vitamin D or could be considered insufficient on the basis of their serum 25(OH)D concentrations.

"We showed that girls who were vitamin D deficient have lower cortical bone density and higher parathyroid hormone concentrations, results that are consistent with secondary hyperparathyroidism," the researchers continued. "Limited exposure to sunlight and low dietary vitamin D intake are the main reasons for vitamin D deficiency during the winter. Our results suggest that vitamin D supplements on an individual basis or through the food supply is indicated for early pubertal and prepubertal girls."

5.

Vitamin D and Seniors

Randomized trials using the currently recommended intakes of 400 IU/day of vitamin D have shown no appreciable reduction in fracture risk, reported Reinhold Vieth of the University of Toronto in Canada and colleagues in various countries.[1]

By contrast, trials using 700–800 IU/day of the vitamin found less fracture incidence, with and without supplemental calcium. The researchers added that the reduction in fracture incidence occurs when blood levels of the vitamin exceed 72 nmol/l, and this change may result from both improved bone health and a reduction in falls due to greater muscle strength, according to Heike A. Bischoff-Ferrari and colleagues, writing in the *American Journal of Clinical Nutrition*.[2]

"Evaluation of most relations of health and disease that involve vitamin D levels lead to the conclusion that a desirable 25(OH)D concentration is over 75 nmol/l (30 ng/ml)," Vieth and colleagues said. "If a concentration of 75 nmol/l is the goal to be achieved by consumption of vitamin D, then why is it so rare for members of the population to accomplish this? One reason is that almost every time the public media report that vitamin D nutrition status is too low or that higher vitamin D intakes may improve health, the advice that accompanies the report is outdated and thus misleading."

Vieth and colleagues go on to say that media reports to the public are typically accompanied by a paragraph that approximates the following: "Current recommendations from the Institute of Medicine call for 200 IU/day from birth through age 50; 400 IU for those 51 to 70; and 600 IU for those over 70. Some experts say that optimal amounts are close to 1,000 IU/day. Until more is known, it is not wise to overdo it." The only conclusion that the public can draw from this is to do nothing different from what they have done in the past, Vieth and colleagues said.

"Regrettably, we are stuck in a revolving cycle of publications that are documenting the same vitamin D inadequacy," the researchers continued. "This phenomenon has been referred to as 'circular epidemiology' and for vitamin D, the phenomenon will continue for as long as the levels of vitamin D fortification and supplementation and the practical advice offered to the public remain essentially the same as they were in the era before we knew that 25(OH)D even existed."

As scientists, the purpose of their work is to improve the health of the public, Vieth and colleagues added. They know the realities of serum 25(OH)D concentrations of populations around the world, and they have come to the conclusion that public health will benefit from improved vitamin D nutritional status.

"We know the intakes of vitamin D needed to bring about desirable 25(OH)D concentrations, so why is the science not making a difference to public health?" they added. "A major reason is that there is little public pressure on policymakers to support efforts to update recommendations about nutrition. Public pressure is generally rooted in the media, but we do not think that the public media present the vitamin D story in a complete and accurate manner."

Supplemental intakes of 400 IU/day of vitamin D have only a modest effect on blood levels of 25(OH)D, which raise them by 7–12 nmol/l, depending on the starting point, Vieth and colleagues said. To raise 25(OH)D from 50 to 80 nmol/l requires an additional intake of around 1,700 IU.

"Safety is the first priority when giving advice to increase supplemental or fortification with any nutrient," the researchers continued.

A recent review applied the risk assessment method used by the Food and Nutrition Board to update the safe, tolerable upper intake level for vitamin D. The method focuses on the risk of hypercalcemia, according to J. N. Hathcock and colleagues.[3]

Hathcock and colleagues added that the conclusion was that the upper limit for vitamin D consumption by adults should be 10,000 IU/day, which indicates that the margin of safety for vitamin D consumption for adults is more than ten times any current recommended intakes.

In addition to Reinhold Vieth, the rather caustic editorial was sanctioned by Michael F. Holick, Bess Dawson-Hughes, Robert P. Heaney, Walter C. Willett, Heike Bischoff-Ferrari, Barbara J. Boucher, Cedric F. Garland, Bruce W. Hollis, Christel Lamberg-Allardt, John J. McGrath, Anthony W. Norman, Robert Scragg, Susan J. Whiting, and Armin Zittermann—all international experts on vitamin D.

In an article in the *American Journal of Nutrition,* Paul F. Jacques of Tufts University in Boston, and colleagues at other facilities, reported that J. L. Omdahl et al. first documented a high prevalence of inadequate vitamin D concentrations in a sample of healthy older Americans from the New Mexico Aging Process Study in 1982. They observed that plasma 25(OH)D concentrations were significantly lower in the elderly—mean 38 nmol/l—than in younger people (73 nmol/l).[4, 5]

"Inadequate vitamin D might be expected to be less frequent in the United States, where milk is supplemented with vitamin D, than in countries where milk is not supplemented," Jacques and colleagues said. "In fact, inadequate vitamin D levels were found to be common among older populations in Britain, Ireland, Switzerland, the Netherlands, Denmark, France, and Spain. A study of older people from 11 European countries found that 36 percent of men and 47 percent of women had vitamin D levels that were less than 30 nmol/l."

In their study, Jacques et al. evaluated blood levels of 25-hydroxyvitamin D concentrations and risk factors for low [25(OH)D] in 290 men and 469 women, ranging in age from sixty-seven to ninety-five, who were in the famous Framingham Heart Study cohort.

In the women, concentrations were inversely associated with age and positively associated with supplemental vitamin D intake and residence in Florida, California, and Arizona; in men they were positively associated with serum creatinine concentrations. Results from the population-based sample of elderly people suggest that inadequate vitamin D status is an important public health problem, which could be readily addressed by adequate vitamin D intake or sunlight exposure, the researchers added.

In their study, only 1 percent of the volunteers with reported intakes of vitamin D over 400 IU/day had concentrations less than 25 nmol/l, and 2.5 percent had concentrations less than 37.5 nmol/l. This confirms the observations of A. R. Webb and colleagues that elderly people who took a vitamin supplement or drank two to three glasses of milk a day were vitamin D–sufficient.[6]

"We found that 75 percent of the women and 80 percent of the men in our population based sample of elderly people did not regularly take vitamin D supplements and, among these unsupplemented people, 68 percent of the women and 64 percent of the men consumed less than 8 oz (240 ml/day) of milk," Jacques and colleagues said. "Obvious dietary improvements could readily increase circulating 25(OH)D concentrations in elderly Americans."

A new study from Wake Forest University in Winston-Salem, North Carolina, suggests that a shortage of vitamin D may play a role in poor physical performance among the elderly, as reported the May 1, 2007, issue of the *New York Times*. The research team, headed by Denise K. Houston, utilized data from an Italian study in which over nine hundred people, sixty-five years of age and older, were tested for vitamin D levels and then asked to perform several tasks, such as walking fast, quickly getting out of a chair, and balancing.[7]

The original study, which appeared in the April 2007 issue of the *Journal of Gerontology,* suggested that people with low levels of vitamin D in their blood did worse on tests involving physical skills. It also confirmed that older people who take vitamin D supplements appear to have gained strength.

Cross-sectional studies show that elderly people with higher intakes of vitamin D in their blood have increased muscle strength and a lower number of falls, according to a study reported the *Journal of Bone and Mineral Health.*[8]

In a double-blind, randomized, controlled trial, a research team at the Prince of Wales Hospital and the Chinese University of Hong Kong evaluated 122 elderly women, sixty-three to ninety-nine years of age, who were in geriatric care.

The volunteers were given 1,200 mg of calcium and 800 IU of cholecalciferol (vitamin D_3) or 1,200 mg of calcium daily during a twelve-week trial. During that time, the number of falls per person was compared between the treatment groups. Among the patients given calcium and vitamin D, there were significant increases in median serum 25-hydroxyvitamin D and 1,25-dihydroxyvitamin D. Before the study began, mean observed number of falls per person per week were 0.059 in the calcium plus vitamin D group and 0.056 in the calcium only group.

During the twelve-week treatment period, mean number of falls per person per week was 0.034 in the calcium and vitamin D group and 0.076 in the calcium group. After adjustment for variables, calcium plus vitamin D treatment accounted for a 49 percent reduction in falls. Among fallers in the treatment group, the average number of falls was significantly higher in the calcium-only group.

In addition, musculoskeletal function improved significantly in the calcium–vitamin D group, the researchers added. A single intervention with vitamin D and calcium over a three-month period reduced the risk of falling by 49 percent, compared with calcium alone. The impact of vitamin D on falls might be explained by the improvement in musculoskeletal function.

A study at Hôpital Edouard Herriot in Lyon, France, headed by Marie C. Chapuy, PhD, evaluated the effect of vitamin D_3 at 20 mcg (800 IU/day) and tricalcium phosphate containing 1.2 g of elemental calcium in 1,634 women, compared to 1,636 women who were given a double placebo.[9]

In the women who completed the eighteen-month study, the number of hip fractures was 43 percent lower and the total number of nonvertebral fractures was 32 percent lower among the patients treated with vitamin D_3 and calcium when compared with those who took the placebo.

In the vitamin D_3–calcium group, mean serum parathyroid hormone concentrations were reduced by 44 percent from baseline—beginning of the study—at the end of eighteen months, and blood concentrations of 25(OH)D had increased 162 percent over baseline.

The research team added that the bone density of the proximal femur (nearest the trunk) increased 2.7 percent in the vitamin D–calcium group and decreased 4.6 percent in the controls. They concluded that vitamin D and calcium supplementation reduce the risk of hip fractures and nonvertebral fractures in elderly women, who had a mean age of eighty-four years.

Hip fractures are the most frequently occurring skeletal problem in developing countries, and they account for nearly 10 percent of all acute surgical beds in Finland, reported Robert P. Heaney, MD, of Creighton University in Omaha, Nebraska. This costs Western nations in the range of $8–20 million U.S. per population (in 1992). These figures will increase as the population gets older, he added.[10]

The two main sites of hip fractures are the intertrochanteric region (two of the bony prominences in the femur) and across the femoral neck. Low bone mass, often found in the elderly, is a risk factor. Also, low vitamin D levels increase the risk of fractures, he said.

Other risk factors include low protein intake, low calcium intake, increased calcium excretion, and osteomalacias superimposed on preexisting bone loss. The researcher suggests that aggressive supplementation, especially with protein, provides substantial hope for improved recovery following a fracture.

In evaluating 747 men with average age of sixty-seven, low intakes of vitamin D were linked with the highest levels of lead in bone, reported the *American Journal of Epidemiology*.[11]

In addition, low intakes of vitamin C and iron revealed the greatest amounts of lead in the bloodstream. The lead-reducing benefits of these nutrients were found to plateau at higher levels of daily consumption, suggesting that vitamins are limited in their ability to fight environmental exposure to lead.

As reported in the *Medical Journal of Australia,* a research team at St. George

Hospital, Kogarah, New South Wales, Australia, evaluated forty-one men, sixty years of age and older, with hip fractures, along with forty-one hospitalized inpatients and fifty-one outpatient controls without hip fractures.[12]

No differences were found between the hip fracture group and the two control groups with regard to osteoporotic hip fractures. Men with the fractures had low mean serum 25-hydroxyvitamin D concentrations when compared to both inpatient and outpatient controls.

The researchers added that subclinical vitamin D deficiency was 63 percent in the fracture group, compared with 25 percent in the controls combined. Also, inpatients with and without hip fractures had significantly lower mean serum albumin, calcium, and free testosterone concentrations than the outpatients. In a multiple regression analysis, subclinical vitamin D deficiency was the strongest predictor of hip fracture. *Subclinical* suggests the presence of a disease without manifest symptoms. This indicates an early step in the progression of the disease, the researchers said.

In the SENECA study of European elderly, eighty to eighty-five years of age, vitamin deficiency was found in 47 percent for vitamin D; 23.3 percent for vitamin B_6; 2.7 percent for vitamin B_{12}; and 1.1 percent for vitamin E.[13]

With aging, there is a reduction in the energy requirement, due to a reduction in lean body mass and a reduction in physical activity, which leads to reduced macro- and micronutritional intake of about 30 percent by eighty years of age, according to the *International Journal of Vitamin and Nutrition Research*.

As reported in the *American Journal of Clinical Nutrition,* researchers evaluated 682 women, sixty-five years of age or older, in the Women's Health and Aging Study I; these women had various health difficulties. Between 6.2 percent and 12.6 percent had a vitamin D deficiency.[14]

The researchers said that a vitamin D deficiency is a common and important public health problem for older disabled women, especially black women. A deficiency in the vitamin is associated with a higher level of disability; however, it can be prevented, although it probably necessitates supplementation beyond that found in milk and cereal, the researchers added.

At Union Memorial Hospital in Baltimore, 244 people sixty-five years of age, of which 116 had been confined indoors for at least six months, were compared with 128 controls. The sunlight-deprived people, of which 54 percent were community dwellers and 38 percent nursing home residents, had blood levels of 25-hydroxyvitamin D below the normal range. The mean intake of the vitamin was 121 IU and 583 mg for calcium, which were below the recommended dietary allowances.[15]

In spite of vitamin D supplementation in foods, there are many elderly people who are confined indoors and who have low vitamin D stores, reported F. Michael Gloth III, MD, and colleagues. This puts them at risk for bone loss, pain, weakness, and subsequent functional impairment. He added that vitamin D supplementation at greater than the RDA could improve vitamin D status in housebound elderly.

In a review of 117 studies on vitamin D from 1971 to 1990, a research team at St. Michael's Hospital in Dublin, Ireland, found that vitamin D fortification or supplementation is necessary to maintain optimal amounts of the fat-soluble vitamin in the elderly.[16]

The researchers, reporting in the *American Journal of Medicine,* said that, while exposure to summer sun is critical in providing vitamin D, oral intake combined with either fortified foods or supplements is essential for maintaining proper tissue stores of the vitamin. Vitamin D intakes are, of course, lower during winter months, when the elderly wear clothes that prevent the formation of vitamin D on their skin.

Aging interferes with the metabolism of vitamin D and calcium, and there is an age-related decline in the skin production of 7-dehydrocholesterol, the precursor of previtamin D_3, according to Norman H. Bell of the Ralph H. Johnson Medical Center in Charleston, South Carolina. Synthesis of vitamin D_3 on the skin is, therefore, reduced.[17]

The intake of vitamin D from exposure to the sun, especially among the housebound or institutionalized elderly, kidney production of 1,25-dihydroxyvitamin D, intestinal absorption of calcium, and the ability to adapt to a low-calcium diet—all these may be reduced in seniors. Researchers have also found a decline in the concentration of vitamin D receptors in the intestinal mucosa of elderly women. Secondary hyperparathyroidism may result with aging and may increase the risk of bone loss, Bell continued.

He went on to say that postmenopausal osteoporosis is related to estrogen deficiency and this tends to occur earlier, between the ages of fifty-one and sixty-five, than senile (age-related) osteoporosis.

In a double-blind, two-year study of 348 postmenopausal women, seventy and older, in the Netherlands, researchers discovered that, compared with placebo, 400 IU/day of vitamin D_3 increased bone mineral density of the femoral neck. No side effects were recorded.

Vitamin D_3 significantly increased blood levels of 25-hydroxyvitamin D and serum 1,25-dihydroxyvitamin D, lowered serum immunoreactive parathyroid hormone, and increased the urinary calcium/creatinine ratio. The study suggested that most of the people were depleted of vitamin D, and that vitamin D_3 increased bone mineral density by correcting the depletion and the secondary hyperthyroidism.

In larger studies of nursing home– or apartment house–based postmenopausal, ambulatory women, 800 IU of vitamin D_3 and 1,200 mg of elemental calcium, given daily for eighteen months, reduced the incidence of hip fractures by 43 percent and nonvertebral fractures by 32 percent, compared with no treatment during the final six months of treatment.

In another study, annual intramuscular injection of vitamin D_2, at 150,000–300,000 IU in one dose, reduced the incidence of fractures in elderly Finnish men and women, and D_3 reduced the incidence of vertebral crush features in Japanese women with senile osteoporosis.

Bell and his colleagues concluded that alterations in vitamin D metabolism and nutrition, which may be prominent in the aging population, may play a significant role in the pathogenesis of senile osteoporosis. Therefore, treatment with vitamin D and its analogs in modest doses may, in certain cases, prevent the loss of bone mass and fractures in the elderly.

In the elderly, reduced exposure to sunlight may be associated with a reduction in vitamin D, and reduced food intake in the elderly may be further compromised by drugs that impair appetite and absorption of vitamin D, vitamin A, vitamin B_1, vitamin B_6, vitamin B_{12}, and vitamin C, according to a study published in the *International Journal of Vitamin and Nutrition Research.* In addition, anticonvulsant drugs and medicines that induce kidney microsomal enzyme activity accelerate vitamin D metabolism and can aggravate postmenopausal bone loss.[18]

As reported in the *British Medical Journal,* a study was conducted involving 3,270 mobile elderly women (mean age of eighty-four), who were living in 180 nursing homes. Half of the women were given 1.2 g/day (1,200 mg) of calcium in the form of tricalcium phosphate, along with 800 IU (20 mcg) of cholecalciferol (vitamin D_3). The others were given a placebo.[19]

Following thirty-six months of follow-up, the likelihood of hip fractures and nonvertebral injury was reduced in the treatment group by 29 percent and 24 percent, respectively. The odds ratio for the reduction in risk of hip fracture was 0.70 and for all nonvertebral fractures 0.70 as well.

The research team, headed by Marie C. Chapuy, PhD, added that there were 17.2 percent fewer women with one or more nonvertebral fractures and 23 percent fewer volunteers with one hip fracture in the treatment group. Also, there was a reduction in the likelihood of hip fractures and all nonvertebral fractures in the treatment group.

In the women who had elevated serum parathyroid concentrations and low vitamin D levels at the beginning of the study, these were normalized after three years of treatment, in contrast to the placebo group, in which the parathyroid hormone levels significantly increased from baseline readings and vitamin D levels remained low. It was also reported that at baseline—beginning of the study—there was a significant correlation between density and serum parathyroid hormone in the 128 women who were evaluated.

According to Ailsa Goulding, PhD, the reasons for increasing vitamin D intake in the elderly include: (1) significant evidence indicates that low vitamin D levels are common in the elderly; (2) modest reductions in blood levels of 25-hydroxyvitamin D stimulate secretion of parathyroid hormone and increase the rate of breakdown of bone and bone loss; (3) plasma 25-hydroxyvitamin D concentrations are correlated strongly with hip bone density in the general community; (4) patients with hip fractures have lower 25-hydroxyvitamin D levels than the controls; and (5) vitamin D and calcium supplements can improve bone density.[20]

Goulding added that fracture risk for those living in institutions has been shown to be 10.5 times higher than for those living independently. Doses at 800 IU/day of vitamin D and 1,200 mg/day of calcium have been shown to reduce fracture rates.

In addition, vitamin D at 700 IU/day and 500 mg/day of calcium improved bone density and reduced nonvertebral bone fractures. It was also reported that injections of vitamin D_2 at 150,000 IU alone have been shown to lower hip fracture risk. Vitamin D supplementation is inexpensive, and oral doses up to 800 IU/day are safe, Goulding reported in the *New Zealand Medical Journal.*

As an elderly person's life expectancy grows and a disease burden accumulates, concern about maintaining functional independence becomes paramount, explained Joseph R. Sharkey, Texas A&M University, College Station, Texas, and colleagues in Florida and North Carolina. In light of these concerns, families, caregivers, health care providers, and home- and community-based providers share the burden of the consequences of an elderly person's disability.[21]

Nutritional intake has often been overlooked as a possible contributing factor to lower-extremity physical performance, especially in homebound elderly, so the objective of their study was to examine the association of calcium, vitamin D, magnesium, and phosphorus intakes with the inability to carry out lower-extremity physical performance tests.

Among the 321 volunteers, age, ethnicity, race, body mass index, arthritis, frequent fear of falling, and lowest SMN (summary musculoskeletal nutrient) intake were independently associated with being unable to perform functional tests. The lowest SMN intake and the highest bone mineral index were significantly associated with increasingly worse levels of lower-extremity performance after adjusting for health and demographic characteristics, they reported in the *American Journal of Clinical Nutrition.*

"Considering the importance of identifying short- and long-term outcomes that help elderly people maintain adequate nutritional status, while remaining independent and at home, the results of our study suggest the need to explore strategies that target the improvement of dietary intake and physical performance," the researchers said.

The importance of vitamin D for bone health and muscle function has long been acknowledged, and accumulating evidence suggests that adequate vitamin D status may contribute to the prevention of autoimmune diseases, high blood pressure, and various types of cancer, reported Rob M. van Dam of Vrije Universiteit Amsterdam in the Netherlands and colleagues in the United States and the Netherlands.[22, 23]

The van Dam study was based on cross-sectional data from white men and women, aged sixty to eighty-seven, who participated in the 2000–2001 Hoorn Study follow-up examination, which was a population-based study of glucose metabolism that started in 1989 and involved people living in the town of Hoorn.

Inadequate vitamin D status can be subdivided into *vitamin D insufficiency,* characterized by elevated serum parathyroid concentrations or a mild increase in bone turnover, and *vitamin D deficiency,* characterized by high bone turnover and possible bone mineralization defects, the researchers explained in the *American Journal of Clinical Nutrition.* Vitamin D insufficiency is highly prevalent in many populations around the world, and vitamin D deficiency is common in institutionalized elderly and Europeans of non-Western origin.

This was a cross-sectional study involving 538 white Dutch men and women, and vitamin D was assessed by blood levels of 25-hydroxyvitamin D (25(OH)D) concentrations. In the winter months, 51 percent of the subjects had blood levels of vitamin D less than 50 nmol/l. Increased body fatness and less time spent on outdoor physical activity were associated with worse vitamin D status.

Regular intake of vitamin D–fortified margarine products, fatty fish, and vitamin D–containing supplements, as opposed to consumption of none of these, was inversely associated with vitamin D inadequacy. The researchers estimated that combined intake of vitamin D–fortified margarine products (20 g/day), fatty fish (100 g/week), and vitamin D supplements, was associated with a 16.8 nmol/l higher vitamin D concentration than was the use of none of these. However, none of the volunteers reached these intakes for all three factors.

"Our findings suggest that increased adiposity and a sedentary lifestyle, which result in less participation in outdoor activities, may contribute to poor vitamin D status," the researchers continued. "Because few foods are vitamin D fortified and amounts of vitamin D in supplements are low, it is difficult to achieve adequate vitamin D through increasing intakes in the Netherlands and countries with similar health policies."

They added that the use of supplements with higher vitamin D doses would be an effective measure for specific high-risk groups, but the experience from campaigns recommending folic acid supplements—the B vitamin—suggest that this strategy may not be effective for large numbers of the general population.

They went on to say that their results indicate that fortification of margarine with vitamin D substantially contributes to better vitamin D status in the Netherlands and that fortification of other widely used foods—milk, yogurt, orange juice, and cereal products—should be considered in those countries where fortification is not currently in vogue.

Patients with a history of falling and vitamin D insufficiency, living in a sunny climate, can benefit from ergocalciferol (vitamin D_2) supplementation in addition to calcium intake, reported the *Archives of Internal Medicine*.[24]

This procedure is associated with a 19 percent reduction in the relative risk of falling, especially in the winter months, the researchers said.

The one-year study involved 302 older women, ranging in age from seventy to eighty, living in Perth, Australia. They had a blood 25-hydroxyvitamin D concentration of less than 24.0 ng/dl and a history of falling.

The participants were given 1,000 IU/day of vitamin D_2, while controls received a placebo. Both groups were given 1,000 mg/day of calcium citrate.

6.

Healthy Bones

Bone is the structural material of the body's framework, or skeleton, reported the *American Medical Association Home Medical Encyclopedia*. It contains calcium and phosphorus, making it hard and rigid. The arrangement of bone fibers makes the bone resilient.[1]

The surface of bone is covered with periosteum, which is a thin membrane that contains a network of blood vessels and nerves. Under the periosteum is a hard, dense shell of compact or ivory bone. Inside this shell, the bone is cancellous or spongy. The central cavity of hollow bones and the meshes of spongy bone contain a fatty tissue (bone marrow), in which red and most white blood cells and platelets are formed.

"The hard, structural part of bone under the periosteum is formed of columns of bone cells known as haversian canals," the publication said. "These are important for the nutrition, growth, and repair of the bone. The direction of the canals corresponds with the mechanical forces acting on the bone. Bone is insensitive and any sensation comes from the nerves in the periosteum."

The long, short, flat, and irregular bones of the skeleton provide a rigid framework for the muscles. The muscles form surface coverings of the cavities that protect the body's organs—the heart and lungs in the bony thoracic cavity, and the brain in the skull. Bones, with joints and muscles, form the locomotor system, the publication continued.

"The growth of bone is a balance between the activity of 2 constituent cells, the osteoblasts and the osteoclasts," the publication said. "Osteoblasts encourage the deposit of the mineral calcium phosphate on the protein framework of the bone. Osteoclasts remove mineral from the bone. The actions of these cells are controlled by hormones: growth hormones, secreted by the pituitary gland, sex hormones, estrogen and testosterone, the adrenal hormones, parathyroid hormones, and the thyroid hormone thyrocalcitonin. These hormones also maintain the calcium level in the blood within close limits. For example, any fall below the normal range affects the nerves and muscles."

Most bones develop in the embryo during the fifth and sixth week of pregnancy, taking the form of cartilage. This cartilage begins to be replaced by hard bone in a process called ossification, at around the seventh or eighth week of gestation. This process is not completed until early adulthood.

At birth, many bones consist mainly of cartilage, which will ossify later. The ends of the long bones are separate from the shaft, which allow the bones to grow. Some small bones of the hands and feet consist entirely of cartilage. Many of the bones of the skull do not begin life as bone. They are called membranous bones.

Bone disorders are investigated by x-rays, CT scanning, and radionuclide scanning, by biopsy, and by biochemical blood tests to look for any abnormalities in the levels of hormones or nutrients, such as calcium and vitamin D, the publication added.

The strength of bone is determined by its material composition and structure, and bone must be stiff and able to resist deformation, thereby making loading possible, explained Ego Seeman, MD, and Pierre D. Delmas, MD, of the University of Melbourne, Australia, in the May 25, 2006, issue of the *New England Journal of Medicine.* Bone must also be flexible and it must be able to absorb energy by deforming, to shorten and widen when compressed and to lengthen and narrow in tension without cracking.[2]

If bone is brittle—too stiff and unable to deform a little—the energy imposed by loading will be released by structural failure, initially by the development of microcracks and then by complete fracture, the researchers said. If bone is too flexible and deforms beyond its peak strain, it will also crack. Bone must also be light enough to facilitate movement.

"Bone is composed of type 1 collagen stiffened by crystals of calcium hydroxyapatite," the researchers added. "An increase in tissue mineral density increases the stiffness of the fabric, but sacrifices flexibility. Human bone is about 60 percent mineralized. The composition and degree of collagen cross-linking also influence function."

Hip fractures increase exponentially with age, so that by the ninth decade of life, an estimated one in every three women and one in every six men will have sustained a hip fracture, according to Heike A. Bischoff-Ferrari, MD, MPH, of the Harvard School of Public Health, Boston, and colleagues at other Boston area facilities. With the aging of the population, the number of hip fractures is projected to increase worldwide.[3]

"The consequences of hip fractures are severe, in that 50 percent of older people have permanent functional disability; 15 to 20 percent require long-term nursing home care; and 10 to 20 percent die within one year," the researchers added. "Besides the personal burden, hip fractures are projected to cost the United States an increase from $7.2 billion in 1990 to $16 billion by 2020."

The objective of their study was to estimate the effectiveness of vitamin D supplementation in preventing hip and nonvertebral fractures in older people. In the study, the researchers conducted a systematic review of all English and non-English articles in Medline and other sources from January 1960 to January 2005 and EMBASE from January 1991 to January 2005. Other literature searches were also conducted.

"For both hip and non-vertebral fracture prevention by vitamin D, our pooled results indicated variation between studies that was resolved when low- and high-dose vitamin D (cholecalciferol) trials were pooled separately," the researchers said. "For trials using 700 to 800 IU/day of oral vitamin D, with or without calcium supplementation, we found a significant 26 percent reduction in risk of sustaining hip fracture and a significant 23 percent reduction in risk of sustaining any non-vertebral fracture vs. calcium or placebo."

They added that the pooled risk differences indicated that forty-five people would need to be treated with 700 to 800 IU/day of vitamin D to prevent one person from sustaining a hip fracture, and twenty-seven people would need to be treated to prevent one person from sustaining any nonvertebral fracture. By contrast, 400 IU/day of vitamin D did not appreciably reduce hip or nonvertebral fractures in older people, compared with placebo or calcium.

The research team said there are two physiological explanations for the benefit of vitamin D on fracture risk in older people: (1) the well-described decrease in bone loss in older people; and (2) vitamin D appears to have a beneficial effect on muscle strength and balance, mediated through highly specific receptors in muscle tissue.

"Furthermore," they continued, "vitamin D has been associated with a significant 22 percent reduction in the risk of falling in older individuals. As both bone loss and falls are important risk factors for fractures in older people, it is plausible that vitamin D supplementation in a sufficient dose reduces the risk of fractures in older people."

Calcium supplements or calcium and vitamin D taken in combination may reduce the risk of bone fractures and bone density loss in older patients, assuming the supplements are taken regularly in large doses, reported Nicholas Bakalar in the September 4, 2007, issue of the *New York Times*.[4]

A review of twenty-nine randomized trials involving more than 63,000 men and women over the age of fifty, as published in the August 25, 2007, issue of the *Lancet,* found that the risk for fractures could be reduced 12 percent with the two supplements.

The researchers reported that the fracture risk was reduced by almost one-quarter in the trials in which patients took the supplements conscientiously. The best effect came when the volunteers took 1,200 mg/day of calcium and 800 IU/day of vitamin D. These levels are slightly different from the recommended dietary allowance, which are 1,200 mg/day of calcium for those over fifty, but the RDA for vitamin D for people fifty to seventy is 400 IU/day, and 600 IU/day for those seventy-one and older.

In five trials, those taking vitamin D and calcium supplements had fewer fractures than those given a placebo, reported Anne M. Wolff, RD, and Andrew Wolff, MD, in *Hospital Medicine.* In one study, elderly volunteers given 700 IU/day of vitamin D and 500 mg/day of calcium were less than half as likely as controls to sustain a fracture.[5]

Older skin is less efficient in converting sunlight to vitamin D and 30–49 percent of adults over fifty either are borderline or overly vitamin D–deficient without symptoms, reported a research team at the Bone Research Laboratory at Boston University Medical Center in Massachusetts. They added that it is difficult to achieve adequate vitamin D intake through diet alone.

"Those living in the northern latitudes and older people are more likely to be vitamin D deficient and should take a daily supplement of 400 to 600 IU/day," the Wolffs said.

A total of 119 women younger than seventy years of age, of whom 80 percent were institutionalized, received a one-year treatment with elemental calcium of 0.5 g and vitamin D_3 at 400 IU, taken in a chewable tablet twice daily, or elemental calcium at 0.6 g and vitamin D_3 at 400 IU as one chewable tablet taken twice daily.[6]

At twelve months, results showed that bone mineral density had increased at all sites in the first group, with a statistically significant improvement at the trochanter, and bone mineral density was slightly increased at the femoral neck and slightly decreased at the other sites in the second group. In both groups, 25-hydroxyvitamin D_3 increased significantly, while bone alkaline phosphatase values were reduced in both groups from baseline (beginning of the study) to month six.

Studies of the elderly at University Hospital, Geneva, Switzerland, have shown that calcium and vitamin D supplements can reduce femoral bone loss in institutionalized patients and reduce the incidence of hip fractures. The femur is the long bone of the thigh. Vitamin K deficiency may also pose an increased risk to bone fragility and hip fractures, added Jean-Philippe Bonjour, MD, and colleagues.[7]

Dr. Bonjour said that a reduced protein intake in hospitalized elderly patients was associated with lower femoral neck bone mineral density and poor physical performance. Increasing protein intake from low to normal might increase the plasma level of IgF-I, a growth factor that has a positive effect on bone mass, which decreases in the elderly, they said.

In forty-six patients being seen at a prosthodontic clinic at a school of dentistry for the extraction of several teeth, half of the volunteers took three daily tablets of a supplement that provided a total of 750 mg of calcium and 375 USP units of vitamin D_2.[8]

The researchers reported a significant reduction in the severity of alveolar bone resorption in the supplemented group. Mean alveolar bone loss for patients receiving the supplement was 36 percent less than for patients given a look-alike pill.

At Tufts University in Boston, Bess Dawson-Hughes, MD, and colleagues evaluated 176 men and 213 women, sixty-five years of age and older, who took 500 mg of calcium citrate malate and 700 IU of vitamin D_3 (cholecalciferol) per day or a placebo. It was found that a significant difference was shown between the calcium–vitamin D and placebo groups at all skeletal sites after one year of therapy. However, the data was only significant for total bone mineral density in the second and third years.[9]

Of the thirty-seven patients who had nonvertebral fractures, twenty-six were in the placebo group and eleven were in the calcium–vitamin D group. In the latter group, there was increased bone density of 0.5 percent, compared with −0.7 percent in the femoral neck; a positive 2.12 percent compared to a positive 1.22 percent of the spine and a total body increase in bone density of 0.006 percent versus −1.09 percent in the placebo group.

Writing in the *American Journal of Clinical Nutrition* in 2002, Dawson-Hughes and Susan S. Harris, discussed their study to determine if supplemental calcium citrate malate and vitamin D influence protein intake and changes in bone mineral density. Protein intake was assessed at midpoint of the study using a food frequency questionnaire and bone mineral density was determined every six months using dual energy x-ray absorptiometry.[10]

Their study initially involved 161 healthy men and 181 healthy women over age sixty-five, who participated in a three-year randomized, placebo-controlled trial, although some of the volunteers dropped out for various reasons.

Those remaining in the study were randomly assigned to receive either 500 mg of calcium citrate malate and 700 IU of vitamin D daily or a double placebo. The volunteers came to the Nutrition Center at Tufts University every six months for bone mineral density and other measurements.

The researchers reported a positive association between dietary protein intake and change in total-body and femoral neck bone mineral density in healthy older men and women who were supplemented with the two nutrients. It did not matter whether the protein came from an animal or a plant source.

"The present study suggests that bone mineral density may be improved by increasing protein intake in many older men and women, as long as they meet the currently recommended intakes of calcium and vitamin D," the researchers concluded.

A debate erupted in the May 25, 2006, issue of the *New England Journal of Medicine,* when a number of letter writers took exception with several conclusions by R. D. Jackson et al. in an earlier issue,[11] who reported that supplemental calcium carbonate increased kidney stones in those participating in the study. There were other bones of contention.

It prompted Susan Terris, MD, PhD, of Red Bank, New Jersey, to comment that the problem might have been avoided if calcium citrate had been used.[12]

Jackson and colleagues also said that calcium and vitamin D reduced the incidence of hip fracture more in older patients than in younger ones. This is not unexpected, Terris said, given the pathophysiological differences between perimenopausal bone loss and senile bone loss. Also, measurement of parathyroid hormone levels to assess the adequacy of vitamin D intake might have helped in the interpretation of their findings. She added that the dose of vitamin D used in the study may have been too low to have had a more dramatic effect in either age group.

Gerson T. Lesser, MD, of Mount Sinai School of Medicine in New York, mentioned that Jackson et al. stated that calcium plus vitamin D did not significantly reduce fracture rates among women fifty to seventy-nine; however, since it has been well-established that bone mineral density decreases progressively in postmenopausal women who are not treated for bone loss, one is struck by the authors' findings that the mean bone mineral density for the total spine and the whole body in the controls increased steadily over the nine years of the study and that bone mineral density for the total hip remained essentially unchanged.[13]

"This phenomenon was surely influenced by the large proportion of controls who were already taking calcium or vitamin D at therapeutic doses," Lesser added. "One would expect improved bone mineral density to be associated with fewer fractures and the investigators did, in fact, find fracture rates for both controls and treated patients to be less than half the rate historically anticipated."

Lesser went on to say that it is also not surprising that the administration of additional calcium and vitamin D–treated subjects further reduced hip fractures only to a limited degree, particularly since the optimal intakes of both nutrients are unknown.

Added Dawson-Hughes of Tufts University in Boston, the results of the Women's Health Initiative trial of calcium and vitamin D (1,000 mg/day of calcium carbonate and 400 IU/day of vitamin D) did not lower fracture rates but did increase the risk of kidney stones in calcium-replete postmenopausal women (mean intake of 1,150 mg/day), whose intake of vitamin D was insufficient.[14]

She said these recommendations should have no effect on the evidence-based recommendation that postmenopausal women, who typically consume 600 mg/day of elemental calcium, should increase their calcium intake to 1,200 mg/day. Similarly, the results should not deter physicians from recommending 800 IU/day of vitamin D—the amount the average postmenopausal woman needs to raise her serum 25-hydroxyvitamin D level to that needed to lower the risk of fracture.

"Finally," she concluded, "the increased risk of kidney stones among the women in the study who were consuming a mean of 2,150 mg/day of calcium—usual mean intake plus supplement—as compared with those consuming 1,150 mg/day, should not be assumed to apply to women who increase their intake to 1,200 mg/day. It is important that the WHI trial not be used to sanction the inadequate intake of calcium and vitamin D that is so widespread among postmenopausal women today."

7.

Amyotrophic
Lateral Sclerosis

Often called Lou Gehrig's disease, amyotrophic lateral sclerosis (ALS) is one of the motor neuron diseases in which the nerves that control muscular activity degenerate inside the brain and spinal cord, reported the *American Medical Association Home Medical Encyclopedia*. This results in weakness and wasting of the muscles.[1]

About one or two cases of ALS are diagnosed in the United States per 100,000 people. This disorder affects people over fifty, and it is more common in men than in women. About 10 percent of the cases are inherited.

In ALS, patients initially notice weakness in the hands and arms, accompanied by atrophy of the muscles. An involuntary quavering of small areas of the muscles may occur. Patients often complain of cramping and stiffness. The weakness may begin in the legs, but all extremities are eventually involved.

The weakness often progresses to muscles of respiration and swallowing, often leading to death in two to four years. However, some patients have lived for over twenty years after diagnosis. Although the patient is unable to speak, swallow, or move, awareness and intellect remain intact.

Henry Louis (Lou) Gehrig (1903–1941) was one of baseball's greatest hitters. He played 2,130 consecutive games—from 1925 to 1939—as a left-handed-hitting first baseman for the New York Yankees. This record was not broken until 1995 by Cal Ripken Jr. of the Baltimore Orioles. In 1939, Gehrig learned that he had ALS.[2]

In eleven patients with Lou Gehrig's disease, blood levels of 25-hydroxyvitamin D were significantly lower than in the controls, as reported in *European Neurology*. Two patients in the study, conducted by Yashihiro Sato and colleagues, had deficient levels, while nine had insufficient amounts of the vitamin.[3]

It was also found that serum parathyroid hormone and ionized calcium levels were elevated in eight and six patients, respectively. Dietary vitamin D intake was below the recommended dietary level of 100 IU/day in ten patients. Two patients lived in a sunlight-deprived area, and Z-scores of mineral bone density and metacarpal index were negative in seven and six patients, respectively.

The research team added that the concentration of vitamin D was positively correlated with the Z-score and negatively correlated with parathyroid hormone levels. Hand-grip dysfunction was correlated with the Z-score of the mineral bone density. They added that there is a disturbance in calcium metabolism, which occurs in a significant number of patients with ALS, according to Sato.

ALS was initially described by the renowned French neurologist Jean-Martin Charcot (1825–1893) of Hôpital Salpetrière in Paris, reported Geoffrey Dean, MD. Charcot observed patients with marked wasting, or atrophy, of the muscles (amyotrophy) and wasting of the nerve fibers in the lateral columns of the spinal cord, causing part of the cord to become hardened or sclerosed. He referred to the disease as *sclerose lateraleamyotrophie*. The French refer to ALS as *la maladie de Charcot* (Charcot's disease). In the United Kingdom, Ireland, and most Commonwealth nations, it is referred to as motor neuron (neurone) disease (MND).[4]

While the cause of ALS is unknown, clues began to surface in 1945, when Harry M. Zimmerman at Montefiore Medical Center and Hospital, Bronx, New York, went to Guam to study medical problems threatening U.S. troops occupying the island, Dean continued. Zimmerman found that ALS, known on the island as lytico, was unusually common among the native Chamorros. In fact, the incidence of ALS was one hundred times greater than had been reported elsewhere in the world. A large number of patients have also been diagnosed with the disease in two villages in the Kii Peninsula in Japan and in some villages in New Guinea.

D. Carleton Gajdusek, a corecipient of the 1976 Nobel Peace Prize in physiology for his work on slow viruses, speculates that the key to the strange disorder in Guam may lie in a mineral imbalance, Dean continued; in particular, a dietary deficiency in calcium and magnesium, coupled with a high intake of aluminum. Researchers have autopsied the brains of ALS patients and have detected abnormally high amounts of aluminum, an anomaly also reported in the brains of patients with Alzheimer's disease.

Stanley Appel, at Baylor College of Medicine in Houston, has found evidence that the sporadic form of ALS may be caused by an excessive influx of calcium into motor neurons, which results in biochemical changes that, ultimately, lead to cell death. The conclusion is that ALS is probably a disorder that has more than one cause.

The aluminum connection and ALS is intriguing, in that the metallic ion is widely distributed in drinking water and soil; it is added to food to make processed food more creamy; and it is widely found in antacids, which have a high aluminum hydroxide content, according to Robert A. Ronzio, PhD.[5]

High levels of aluminum may inhibit phosphate uptake by the intestines and may increase calcium loss by excretion by the kidneys. This imbalance can cause brittle bones and disturb bone formation, Ronzio added.

Aluminum-related diseases include vitamin D–resistant osteomalacia, iron adequate mitocytic anemia, and dialysis dementia, according to R. Bruce Martin of the University of Virginia at Charlottesville. These are three conditions brought about by long-standing hemodialysis.[6]

He added that aluminum is a possible cause of a high frequency of ALS and Parkinson's dementia among the natives of southern Guam, the Kii Peninsula of Japan, and western New Guinea.

Aluminum interferes with the calcium transport system, according to G. B. van der Voet and F. A. Wolff of Leiden University in the Netherlands. Their data suggests that aluminum may mimic calcium in the sodium-dependent intestinal passage.[7]

A number of researchers have speculated that, among those living in the Kii Peninsula in Japan and in Guam, aluminum-related diseases include vitamin D–resistant osteomalacia, iron-adequate microcytic anemia, and dialysis dementia.

Judging by the literature, there is much to learn about ALS and its calcium/vitamin D connection, as well as its relation to other trace minerals.

8.

Cancer

Cancer is an ancient disease, since it was initially identified by Hippocrates and Galen under different names, according to Mukti H. Sarma, PhD. At the end of the nineteenth century, physicians for the first time could diagnose cancer in medical terms. However, only in 1915, after two Japanese researchers, K. Yamagiwa and K. Ichikawa, discovered that continuous application of coal tar to rabbits' skin produced malignancy were experimental studies on cancer initiated.[1]

"Although there are many theories regarding the causes of cancer, the fundamental idea underlying these theories is that the genetic material—the DNA of the cell—has been changed and the various theories attempt to explain how the change was brought about," Sarma said.

The DNA in a cancer cell is slightly different from that of a normal cell, Sarma added. That means that the sequence of the bases—adenine (A), guanine (G), thymine (T), and cytosine (C)—in a given strand of DNA is not the same. These sequences dictate the sequence of the transcribed messenger RNA, which, in turn, specifies the kinds of proteins to be synthesized in a cell. This change in the DNA sequence in the cancer cells results in abnormal proteins, and these new proteins influence the mechanism of growth control in such a way that cell division continues indefinitely.

"The basic change in the DNA—known as mutation—can be caused by many factors, such as ultraviolet and ionizing radiation, chemicals, free radicals, and viruses," Sarma said. "Mutation does not necessarily cause cancer. This only occurs if proteins that result from mutation affect the cellular growth-control mechanism."

Tumors formed from rapidly dividing cells are of two types—benign and malignant, added *Foods & Nutrition Encyclopedia*. Benign tumors are those that cannot invade surrounding tissues and remain strictly local growths. Malignant tumors spread from their original site and can move throughout the body via the bloodstream and the lymphatic system. These cancers are divided into three groups:[2]

1. *Carcinomas* arise in the epithelial tissues, that is, the cells covering the surface of the body and the lining of the glands.

2. *Sarcomas* arise in supporting structures, such as fibrous tissue or connective tissue, and blood vessels.

3. *Leukemias* and *lymphomas* arise in blood-forming cells of the bone marrow and lymph nodes.

Cancers are additionally classified by the organ in which they originate and by the kind of cell involved. Consequently, there are one hundred or more distinct varieties of cancer, such as lung, colon and rectum, breast, larynx, prostate, uterus, kidney, bladder, and so on.

It has been recognized for some time that, apart from its effects on calcium homeostasis, 1,25-dihydroxyvitamin D—$1,25(OH)2D_3$—exhibits potent antiproliferation and differentiating activities, according to Florence Rozen and colleagues at McGill University in Montreal.[3]

While clinical investigation of this antineoplastic activity is limited by the hypercalcemia associated with high doses of vitamin D, novel vitamin D antigens with potent nonproliferative activity but little effect on calcium balance have been described, the researchers said.

The effects of vitamin D and its analogs are modulated by the vitamin D receptor (VDR), which is a member of the nuclear steroid hormone receptor family. VDRs affect gene expression by binding to specific vitamin D response elements in the promoter region of target genes, the researchers continued.

The research team added that their results indicate that vitamin D–related compounds stimulate production of insulinlike growth factor binding protein 5, thereby indirectly suppressing cell proliferation.

As reported in the *American Journal of Clinical Nutrition* in 2007, a research team at Creighton University in Omaha, Nebraska, headed by Joan M. Lappe, conducted a four-year study involving 1,024 women and found that calcium and vitamin D supplements reduced all cancer risk in postmenopausal women. The volunteers were community-dwelling women who were selected from the population of healthy postmenopausal women, over fifty-five years of age, and who resided in a nine-county rural area in Nebraska.[4]

"Our findings of decreased all cancer risk with improved vitamin D status are consistent with a large and still growing body of epidemiological and observational data showing that cancer risk, cancer mortality, or both, are inversely associated with sun exposure, vitamin D status, or both," said Lappe.

The women were randomly assigned to be given either 1,400 mg/day of calcium citrate or 1,500 mg/day of calcium carbonate, plus 1,100 IU/day of vitamin D_3, or a calcium–vitamin D placebo. The researchers found that the risk of cancer was lower in those getting calcium and vitamin D, compared to the controls getting a calcium–vitamin D placebo.

A number of epidemiologic studies suggest that sunlight deprivation, which results in lower levels of vitamin D_3 derivatives, may increase the risk of breast, colon, and prostate cancers, according to researchers at the University of Medicine and Dentistry of New Jersey Medical School in Newark. Pineal function may also be involved. The pineal gland, located in the brain, is responsible for the secretion of the hormone melatonin.[5]

The researchers said that vitamin D derivatives can induce differentiation of several neoplastic cell types, arrest or retard their proliferation, as well as act as chemopreventive agents. Vitamin D_3 is thought to act on several types of tumor progression.

Data suggests that cancers of the breast and prostate act more aggressively in African Americans than in white Americans.

Evidence of vitamin D's protective effect against cancer is compelling, said Bill Sardi in *Nutrition Science News*. For example, research suggests there is a causal relationship with sun exposure that acts through the body's vitamin D metabolic pathways. Some evidence points to a prostate, breast, and colon cancer belt in the United States, which lies in northern latitudes under more cloud cover than other regions during the year, and rates for these cancers are two to three times higher than in sunnier areas.[6]

"Dark skinned people require more sun exposure to make vitamin D," Sardi added. "The thickness of the skin layer called the stratum corneum affects the absorption of UV radiation. Consequently, black human skin is thicker than white skin and thus transmits only about 40 percent of the UV rays for vitamin D production."

He goes on to say that darkly pigmented people who live in sunny equatorial climates experience a higher mortality rate—not incidence—from breast and prostate cancer when they move to geographic areas that are deprived of sunlight during the winter.

At Virginia Polytechnic Institute and State University in Blacksburg, Virginia, a study evaluated 106 adult cancer patients with early stages of active disease for six months or less, but only sixty-two returned dietary questionnaires. Among those who returned the questionnaires, it was found that the patients had substantial dietary deficiencies and probably would have benefited from counseling and/or supplements.[7]

The nutrient intake of male and female cancer patients in the study, compared with those in a Food and Drug Administration survey, was lower in ten vitamins and minerals, including vitamins A, C, D, E, B_1, B_2, B_3, B_6, B_{12}, and the mineral zinc.

BRAIN CANCER

As reported by researchers at the University of Pavia in Italy, two human glioblastoma cell lines were exposed to 25-dihydroxyvitamin D_3 and its metabolite 1-alpha, 25-dihydroxyvitamin D_3. Both substances induced significant reduction—over 50 percent—in the growth of the two glioblastoma cell lines. Glioblastoma multiforme is a fast-growing and highly malignant type of brain tumor. It is a tumor arising from glial (supporting) cells within the brain.[8]

The growth was due to cell death, and the data suggests that, at least in lab glassware, vitamin D metabolites alone or in combination with retinols (vitamin A) may be potential therapies in human malignant gliomas.

BREAST CANCER

In a population-based case control study of 972 women with newly diagnosed breast cancer and 1,135 controls, published in *Cancer Epidemiology Biomarkers and Prevention* in 2007, the results suggest that exposure to sources of vitamin D, especially earlier in life (ten to nineteen years of age), may reduce the risk of breast cancer.[9]

Using logistic regression adjusted for potential cofounders, an inverse association was found between sun exposure from ages ten to nineteen years of age and the risk of breast cancer, where the highest quartile of outdoor activities was associated with a 35 percent reduced risk of breast cancer, compared with the lowest quartile.

Also, cod-liver oil—a rich source of vitamin D—consumed during the period from ten to nineteen years of age was associated with a 24 percent reduced risk of breast cancer. In addition, drinking ten or more glasses of milk—fortified with vitamin D—per week during the period from ten to nineteen years of age, compared with no milk drinking, was associated with a 38 percent reduced risk of breast cancer. (Unfortunately, young girls often avoid milk because of the calories—milk sugar—and the fear of gaining weight.)

The researchers admitted that weaker associations were observed between the exposure to sources of vitamin D from ages twenty to twenty-nine on breast cancer risk, and no associations were reported between exposure to sources of vitamin D from ages forty-five to fifty-four and breast cancer risk.

"We found strong evidence to support the hypothesis that vitamin D could help prevent breast cancer," the researchers said. "However, our results suggest that exposure earlier in life, especially during breast cancer development, may be most relevant," stated Julia A. Knight.

At the 2006 annual meeting of the American Association for Cancer Research, held at Mount Sinai Hospital in Toronto, Canada, Julia A. Knight (just mentioned) suggested that vitamin D exposure early in life may lower a woman's breast cancer risk later in life. The study involved 576 women, twenty to fifty-nine years of age, who had been diagnosed with breast cancer. They were compared to 1,135 healthy, age-matched controls.[10]

Knight reported that sun exposure, including a number of outdoor activities, from ages ten to nineteen and twenty to twenty-nine, along with cod-liver oil consumption—ten years or more—and consumption of ten or more glasses of milk weekly, were found to correlate with a lower risk of breast cancer. The vitamin apparently provides protection against breast cancer as the breast develops during adolescence, Knight said.

A low dietary intake of calcium and vitamin D, coupled with a high intake of phosphorus, might increase women's susceptibility to some forms of breast cancer, according to a research team from the University of Western Ontario in Canada and Memorial Sloan-Kettering Cancer Center in New York.[11]

In the researchers' first study, the combination of calcium, phosphorus, and vitamin D and the development and progression of mammary cancer were evaluated independently. Laboratory animals were fed a semipurified diet, including the carcinogenic chemical DMBA. A week later, the animals were switched to a diet with a special mineral mix that varied in the amount of the two minerals and increased vitamin D from low to high.

The animals were weighed weekly and the mammary glands were monitored at two-week intervals. Results showed that phosphorus and vitamin D had interactive effects with calcium.

In a second study, dietary intake of vitamin D was monitored for its effect on tumorigenesis. The results showed that high intakes of vitamin D inhibited the growth of tumors when calcium and phosphorus intakes were low. The researchers concluded that low intakes of vitamin D and high intakes of phosphorus might reduce calcium bioavailability and increase the risk of breast cancer.

In studying 190 women with breast cancer, compared with a cohort of 5,009 white women who had completed a dermatological exam, several measures of sunlight exposure and dietary vitamin D intake were associated with a reduced risk of breast cancer, according to a study published in *Cancer Epidemiology, Biomarkers and Prevention*.[12]

The researchers said the risk reduction was highest among women who lived in regions of high solar radiation, and there were no risk reductions found among women who lived in regions of low solar radiation.

Vitamin D analogs may offer a potential endocrine therapy for breast cancer, according to James E. Marti. In a study reported in the September 23, 1991, issue of *Cancer Weekly*, women with advanced breast cancer were treated with 1 g/day of calcitriol ointment for six weeks. During that time, 21 percent showed a partial slowing of the spread of cancer. Other studies have reported that colon cancer is less common among those who have high blood levels of vitamin D.[13]

In one study, lasting nineteen years, it was found that daily intake of more than 3.75 mcg of vitamin D reduced the incidence of colon cancer by 50 percent, Marti said. And daily intake of at least 1,200 mg of calcium was said to reduce the risk of colon cancer by 75 percent.

Sunlight or vitamin D may play a protective role in women with breast cancer, reported Susan S. Tomlinson of Union Memorial Hospital in Baltimore. Increasing the intake of fish that contains large amounts of vitamin D—herring, mackerel, salmon, sardines, and the like—may also help to maintain vitamin D levels.[14]

Vitamin D_2 and synthetic D_3 analogs may be beneficial in the endocrine treatment of estrogen receptor-positive and receptor-negative breast cancer. In fact, there may be single-agent treatment with a low calcemic vitamin D_3 analog or with a vitamin D analog that may be used with other tumor-effective drugs, which may be of greater benefit, reported *Physiology, Molecular Biology, and Clinical Applications*. Aside from the calcemic side effects of vitamin D_3

analogs, other negative effects may include immunosuppression and increased risk of bone metastases.[15]

The research team added that vitamin D has an antiproliferation effect, although the mechanism by which it operates is not clear. Vitamin D may suppress breast cancer growth independent of the presence of the estrogen receptor, they added.

Animal studies have suggested that increasing dietary calcium and vitamin D may inhibit the development of breast cancer, according to an article published in the *Journal of the American College of Nutrition.* And epidemiologic studies of breast cancer and exposure to sunlight support the role of vitamin D in the inhibition of breast cancer.[16]

Vitamin D induces differentiation of mammary gland cells, and humans with vitamin D receptor-positive tumors were shown to have a longer disease-free survival than those with receptor-negative tumors, the researchers said.

It was also reported that, in animal models, a Western-type diet with reduced calcium and vitamin D and increased fat induced hyperproliferation and hyperplasia in the mammary gland and colonic epithelium in short-term studies. Dietary calcium supplements inhibited these changes.

The researchers added that studies on osteoporosis resemble those of breast cancer in terms of dietary requirements and recommendations. There is little risk of too much vitamin D unless you take more than 2,000 IU/day (50 mcg), they added.

In an article in *Primary Care and Cancer,* researchers reviewed the concept that inadequate levels of dietary calcium and vitamin D may increase the risk of breast cancer and other types of cancer in young women and the elderly.[17]

Young women generally consume half the recommended levels of calcium in their diets, and this is most likely due to concerns about weight. Dietary deficiencies in calcium and vitamin D during this period of increased epithelial cell proliferation during puberty and adolescence could put girls at an increased risk of breast cancer later in life. It is possible that the mammary gland proliferates during adolescence, the researchers added.

The elderly have low blood circulating levels of 25-hydroxyvitamin D, largely because they are concerned about sun exposure, the researchers continued. Receptors for 1,25-dihydroxyvitamin D, the active form of the vitamin, are present in the pancreas, the brain, and the placenta. Studies have reported that vitamin D analogs suppress the growth of malignant cells without inducing hypocalcemia.

COLON CANCER

A study by Roberd M. Bostick, MD, and colleagues at the University of Minnesota in Minneapolis, evaluated whether or not a high intake of calcium, vitamin D, and dairy products protected against colon cancer. Data was collected from a cohort of 35,215 Iowa women, fifty-five to sixty-nine years of age, who did not have cancer. In four years, 212 colon cancer cases had been diagnosed.[18]

The findings of this study are consistent with the possibility of a 20–30 percent reduction in colon cancer risk with high intakes of calcium, vitamin D, and milk products, the research team reported in the *American Journal of Epidemiology.*

Although the multivariate-adjusted estimates were not statistically significant when considered in the context of the whole body of literature on the subject, the researchers concluded that calcium, vitamin D, and milk products, or some other factors in these foods, may modestly reduce the risk of colon cancer.

In another article in the *American Journal of Epidemiology,* 48,115 American women who were free of colorectal cancer or polyps at the beginning of the trial were followed for twenty-two years. It was found that those with higher intakes of calcium and vitamin D had a reduced risk of distal colorectal adenoma.[19]

The volunteers filled out food frequency questionnaires at the beginning of the study, and the highest quintile of total calcium intake was associated with a 12 percent reduced risk of distal colorectal adenoma and a 27 percent reduced risk of large adenoma, when compared with the lowest quintile of intake.

In addition, the highest quintile of total vitamin D intake was associated with a 21 percent reduced risk of distal colorectal adenoma and a 33 percent reduced risk of distal colon adenoma, compared with the lowest quintile of intake.

The research team added that the combined high intake of vitamin D and low intake of vitamin A (retinol) was associated with a 45 percent reduced risk of distal colorectal adenoma, when compared to low intakes of vitamin D and high intakes of retinol.

The research team concluded that higher total calcium and vitamin D intakes were associated with reduced risk of colorectal cancer and that the actions of vitamin D may be attenuated by high vitamin A intake.

The etiology of colorectal cancer is multifactorial, according to Marcus J. Burnstein, MD, in that it is an interactive complex of fat, fiber, and micronutrients. He is with St. Michael's Hospital in Toronto.[20]

Case-control studies investigating the relation between colorectal cancer and dietary fat consumption have yielded inconsistent results, he added. However, there is an inverse relationship between fiber intake and colorectal cancer. Fibers from fruits and vegetables may have a more protective effect than cereal fibers.

He went on to say that nutrients having a beneficial effect include calcium, selenium, and vitamins A, C, D, and E.

Reporting in the *American Journal of Clinical Nutrition* in 2006, James C. Fleet of Purdue University, West Lafayette, Indiana, commented on an article by E. A. Platz et al. (*Cancer Causes and Control* 11 [2000]: 579–588), who said that over 70 percent of colon cancer risk is preventable through a combination of dietary and lifestyle changes. Other studies have shown that 1,200 mg/day of calcium reduced the risk of advanced colorectal lesions and that calcium-rich dairy foods are also chemoprotective against colon cancer.[21]

Fleet was commenting specifically on an article by S. C. Larsson et al. in the same issue of the *American Journal of Clinical Nutrition*, in which the Larsson study was part of the ongoing Cohort of Swedish Men Trial, which was established in 1997 to study lifestyle/disease interactions. Their study was aimed at determining whether the consumption of different dairy products provides site-specific protection from colon cancer.

A missing feature in their study, Fleet said, is the impact of vitamin D status on the interaction between calcium intake, dairy intake, and colon cancer risk.

"Although many population studies have assessed dietary vitamin D intake, recent evidence suggests that dietary intake does not adequately meet the physiologic needs in certain population subgroups—for example, the elderly and dark skinned people—and geographic regions," Fleet said.

Since dietary vitamin D intake is not the only contributor to vitamin D status, one would need to assess vitamin D status directly, by measuring 25-hydroxyvitamin D concentrations, or at least incorporate estimates of sunlight exposure to determine the contribution of vitamin D to colon cancer risk, he continued.

He went on to say that, given that the interaction between vitamin D status and calcium metabolism is well established, and that vitamin D status appears to modulate the effects of calcium on colon cancer risk, future studies on calcium and dairy intakes and cancer risk should not ignore it.

Writing in the *Journal of the American Medical Association*, Jeffrey A. Meyerhardt, MD, of Dana-Farber Cancer Institute in Boston, and colleagues at various facilities in the United States and Canada, reported that higher intakes of a Western-type diet may be associated with a higher risk of recurrence and mortality among those with stage III colon cancer treated with surgery and adjuvant chemotherapy. Researchers are still trying to identify which components are useful for patients who already have cancer.[22]

"Because ours was an observational study, causality cannot and should not be drawn from these data," Meyerhardt said. "Nonetheless, the data suggests that a diet characterized by higher intakes of red and processed meats, sweets, desserts, french fries, and refined grains increases the risk of cancer occurrence and decreases survival."

The research team added that epidemiological research indicates that dietary factors are associated with the risk of developing colon cancer and that consumption of red meat, alcohol, calcium and vitamin D, vitamin E, and folic acid—the B vitamin—are among the components that appear to influence the risk of developing the disease. Individual components of the diet interact with each other, and confounding can make identification of a specific food or nutrient difficult.

In the February 16, 2006, issue of the *New England Journal of Medicine,* Jean Wactawski-Wende, PhD, and colleagues discussed the Women's Health Initiative (WHI) trial on calcium and vitamin D and the risk of colorectal cancer.[23]

Responding to the article in the May 25, 2006, issue of the journal, Michael F. Holick, MD, PhD, of Boston University Medical Center, said that the chief problem with the study is that, as the authors acknowledged, the dose of 400 IU of vitamin D_3 was inadequate to raise the blood levels of 25-hydroxyvitamin D to what is now considered a healthful range above 30 ng/ml.[24]

"It is now generally recommended that 1,000 IU/day of vitamin D_3 is necessary to attain this level and to maximize intestinal absorption of calcium for optimal bone health and the prevention of cancer," Holick said.

He noted that virtually all the people in the study had vitamin D insufficiency, according to the criterion just given, both at the beginning and at the end of the trial.

"The most important finding in this study is that women in the lowest quartile of serum 25-hydroxyvitamin D levels—less than 31 nmol/liter—had an incidence of colorectal cancer that was 253 percent of the incidence in the highest quartile—serum vitamin D levels more than 58.4 nmol/liter. These women needed more vitamin D," Holick added.

Commenting on the same study, Edward Giovannucci, MD, ScD, of the Harvard School of Public Health in Boston, said that, although the WHI trial provides important data, the benefits of calcium and vitamin D may exist at doses and durations not assessed in the study.[25]

Replying to Drs. Holick and Giovannucci, Jean Wactawski-Wende, PhD, of the University of Buffalo in New York and colleagues at other locations, said that the calcium plus vitamin D intervention trial in the WHI trial was chosen in the early 1990s and that the trial was designed to evaluate the primary effect of supplementation on hip fractures. At the time, 400 IU of vitamin D_3 was considered substantial. Some studies have recommended larger intakes, although there is no current consensus on optimal intake, especially for the prevention of colorectal cancer, she said.[26]

"We believe a better understanding of the discrepancies in the preceding observational studies and in this randomized trial is needed before the role of calcium and vitamin D in the prevention of colorectal cancer can be established," she added.

The debate continued in the November 8, 2007, issue of the magazine when Roger Bouillon, MD, PhD, of Katholieke Universiteit Leuven in Belgium and colleagues in the United States and the Netherlands, agreed with Holick that blood levels of 25-hydroxyvitamin D should exceed 20 ng/ml to avoid bone problems. However, they said, requiring levels above 32 ng/ml implies that over 80 percent of the European population and half of the world population is vitamin D–deficient. They added that data do not support advising pregnant and lactating women that up to 4,000 IU/day of vitamin D is safe.[27]

Robert C. Cava, MD, of Miami Medical Consultants in Coral Gables, Florida, and Andrei Nicole D. Javier of Yale University, in another response, said that the majority of their vitamin D–deficient patients have been treated with 50,000 IU/week of vitamin D for up to two years with no clinical evidence of toxicity or hypercalcemia or elevated blood levels.[28]

Still other researchers, William R. Howe, MD, of the University of Colorado School of Medicine, Aurora, Colorado, and Robert Dellavalle, MD, PhD, of Denver, said that Holick overstates the degree to which sunscreen use reduces levels of vitamin D_3, since few people would apply the large amount of sunscreen that would correlate with the controlled lab tests he references.[29]

"Instead of exposing people to higher levels of a known carcinogen—UV light—dietary vitamin D supplementation and a balanced diet may be a better choice for achieving healthy levels of vitamin D," the two letter writers said.

Still, another writer, Giampiero Igli Baroncelli, MD, of S. Chiara University Hospital, Pisa, Italy, said that Holick reports that for children up to one year ge, who are breastfed without vitamin D supplementation, 400 IU/day of vitamin D prevents vitamin D deficiency. However, the current recommendation by the American Academy of Pediatrics for breastfed infants is 200 IU/day and that this amount can maintain the serum 25-hydroxyvitamin D level at or above 11 ng/ml.[30]

He added that, to his knowledge, there is no evidence of vitamin D deficiency rickets in breastfed infants receiving 200 IU/day of vitamin D, and that vitamin D supplementation to prevent rickets should be efficacious and cost effective.

Holick noted that Bouillon et al. voiced concern about his recommendations concerning vitamin D doses and said that the observations that the maximum calcium transport, lowest parathyroid hormone levels, and greatest muscle strength and bone density occur when 25-hydroxyvitamin D levels are above 30 ng/ml, and that, among women who were given 1,100 IU/day of vitamin D_3 per week, the risk of cancer was reduced by 60 percent.[31]

"Poorly substantiated reports that outbreaks of vitamin D intoxication in the 1950s occurred from the addition of pharmacologic doses of vitamin D to milk have led to unjustified fear in the medical community of inducing vitamin D toxicity," Holick said.

He added that the recommendation to avoid any direct sun exposure because of the risk of skin cancer has resulted in a global pandemic of vitamin D deficiency. In fact, he added, at least half of the European and U.S. populations currently have insufficient levels of vitamin D.

Replying to Cava and Javier, Holick noted that their recommendation of taking 7,000 IU/day of vitamin D_2—versus their 50,000 IU/week—is not a toxic level. A recommendation of 1,000 to 2,000 IU/day of the vitamin is reasonable, as suggested by Norman and colleagues (A. W. Norman et al., "13th Workshop Consensus for Vitamin D Nutritional Guidelines," *Journal of Steroid Biochemistry & Molecular Biology* 103 [2007]: 204–205).

He noted that Howe and Dellavalle questioned the effect of sunscreen in reducing vitamin D synthesis.

"Many sunscreen products have a sun protective factor (SPF) of 30 to 50," Holick continued, "but, even if only 30 percent of the total volume is applied, vitamin D_3 synthesis would be reduced by 95 to 99 percent. One cannot get an adequate amount of vitamin D from a balanced diet alone and, for that reason, supplementation should be recommended."

In replying to Baroncelli's observation concerning the discrepancy between

Holick's recommendation and the American Academy of Pediatrics recommendation, Holick said that it is his hope that the AAP will reconsider the scientific evidence that vitamin D deficiency in childhood is associated with an increased risk of several chronic conditions, as outlined in his review, and might thus revise its recommendation to be equivalent to the Canadian Pediatric Society's current recommendation of 400 IU/day for all neonates.

OVARIAN CANCER

As reported in the *International Journal of Epidemiology*, women have a higher risk of developing ovarian cancer in northern latitudes than they do in southern latitudes, because of a lesser availability of sunshine and vitamin D.[32]

As an example, mortality rates from ovarian cancer were evaluated from the one hundred largest counties in the United States between 1979 and 1988. It was found that ovarian cancer deaths were invariably proportional to mean daily sunshine. This remained after adjusting for variables.

The researchers added that the data should be considered preliminary, and further research using case control and prospective studies are warranted.

PANCREATIC CANCER

A higher vitamin D intake has been associated with a significantly reduced risk of pancreatic cancer, according to Nicholas Bakalar in the September 19, 2006, issue of the *New York Times*. The full study was published in the September 2006 issue of *Cancer Epidemiology, Biomarkers and Prevention*.[33]

The research team at the University of Wisconsin in Madison, headed by Halcyon Skinner, MD, combined data from two prospective studies that involved 46,771 men, ranging in age from forty to seventy-five, and 75,427 women, ranging in age from thirty-eight to sixty-five. During this sixteen-year study, the researchers identified 365 patients with pancreatic cancer.

"After statistically adjusting for age, smoking, level of physical activity, intake of calcium and vitamin A, and other factors, the association between vitamin D intake and reduced risk of pancreatic cancer was still significant," Bakalar said.

For example, compared with patients who consumed less than 150 IU/day of vitamin D, those who consumed more than 600 IU/day reduced their risk by 41 percent.

"It's a promising lead for a disease that has had very few promising leads," Skinner said.

However, the researchers admitted that they did not have definitive information about sun exposure, which also increases production of vitamin D, and they could not exclude the possibility that vitamin D accompanies some other factor that would explain the effect.

ENDOMETRIAL CANCER

Using a database from the World Health Organization, Cedric F. Garland, MD, and colleagues at the University of California at San Diego, found lower rates of endometrial cancer in women with a higher exposure to UV-B radiation, the UV light that helps the skin produce vitamin D, reported the November 27, 2007, issue of the *New York Times*.[34]

The researchers evaluated endometrial cancer—the cancer that affects the lining of the uterus—in patients from 107 countries. They reported that, in both northern and southern hemispheres, the higher the latitude, the higher the risk of the cancer. Obesity was also a risk factor.

"We believe that vitamin D accounts for the finding since the geographic distribution corresponds to that of other cancers which have been shown in studies of individuals to be related to levels of vitamin D," added Garland, whose complete study was published in the November 2007 issue of *Preventive Medicine*.

9.

Cardiovascular Disease

judging by the scientific literature, scientists are just now unraveling vitamin D's impact on cardiovascular disease, coronary heart/artery disease, congestive heart failure, and so forth. In the meantime, of the 71,300,000 American adults with one or more types of cardiovascular disease, 27,400,000 are estimated to be sixty-five or older.

The grim statistics, from the American Heart Association in Dallas, are as follows:[1]

- High blood pressure: 65,000,000. This is defined as systolic (beating) pressure of 140 mm/Hg or greater, and/or diastolic (resting) pressure of 90 mm/Hg or greater.

- Coronary heart disease: 13,200,000; myocardial infarction (heart attack): 7,200,000; and angina pectoris (chest pain): 6,500,000.

- Heart failure: 5,000,000.

- Stroke: 5,500,000.

- One in three adult men and women has some form of cardiovascular disease.

- Coronary heart disease caused one of every five deaths in the United States in 2003.

- Coronary heart disease is the single largest killer of American men and women. Every twenty-six seconds an American will suffer a coronary event, and about every minute someone will die from one.

- Over 83 percent of those who die of coronary heart disease are sixty-five or older.

• The estimated direct and indirect cost for coronary heart disease in 2006 was $142.5 billion.

A great deal of insight as to how vitamin D relates to cardiovascular disease is provided by David S. Grimes, MD, who was interviewed by Kirk Hamilton in *Clinical Pearls*. Grimes was with the Blackburn Royal Infirmary in the United Kingdom.[2]

The northwest of the British Isles, Finland, and the northern part of Sweden have the highest coronary artery disease rates in the world, Grimes said. "It became increasingly clear to me that in Europe there is a 'latitude factor,' since there is a steady gradient of deaths from coronary artery disease with a low level of deaths in the Mediterranean countries, gradually increasing toward the northwest of Europe, with the highest levels in the northwestern parts of the British Isles and northern Scandinavia," Grimes continued.

Analysis has shown that geography plays a fascinating role in this regard, he said. Studies in New Mexico show that living at a high altitude is protective against coronary artery disease. Living at a high altitude and living close to the equator have two things in common—an increase in sunlight and UV exposure. He added that heart disease is common among the poor in Britain, who cannot afford a vacation in the sun, as well as Asians, who have a cultural tendency to avoid the sun.

"The way in which sunlight affects coronary heart disease depends on our vision of the cause of the disease," Grimes added. "For several years, I have been impressed by the idea that coronary heart disease is due to a microbe and that the avoidance of this is increasing all the time. Studies in England have shown that the high incidence of TB in the Asian population appears to be linked to sunlight deficiency and the probability that vitamin D is concerned, not just to bone metabolism, but also to immunocompetence."

He goes on to say that the link suggests that if coronary heart disease is due to microbia—possibly *Chlamydia pneumonia*—then sunlight deficiency would suppress immunity and promote a greater progression of the disease.

"While researching vitamin D," Grimes continued, "I was struck by the chemical similarities between vitamin D and cholesterol, and I realized that they had the same precursor, that is squalene. I had never been comfortable with the basic cholesterol theory. Although a high blood cholesterol is undoubtedly associated with a high coronary risk, the cause of high cholesterol has never been very clear. Once again this has been put down to faulty diet, etc., but this does not seem to work out."

In further studies, he realized that sunlight could determine whether the metabolism of squalene—a precursor of sterols such as cholesterol—went into vitamin D, in the presence of sunshine, or into cholesterol, if sunlight were deficient.

"I, therefore, felt that a high blood cholesterol was a manifestation of sunlight deficiency and I hypothesized that the cholesterol level of blood would be highest in the winter months than in summer, higher with increasing distance from the equator and lower in people with gardens—with a corresponding higher vitamin D level," he said.

Grimes added that we need to recognize that a disease has a single cause and this applies to coronary heart disease. This is reinforced by pathology, and we should not posit that coronary heart disease is due to a genetic factor in one person, smoking in another, faulty diet in another, and so forth.

"I propose that sunlight, acting through vitamin D and enhanced immunity, inhibits the progression of coronary heart disease, and that sunlight deficiency with consequent high cholesterol levels would accelerate the disease and that the pharmaceutical inhibition of cholesterol synthesis would have an inhibiting role," Grimes said.

He suggests that cigarette smoking increases the frequency of respiratory tract infections and that the most common respiratory pathogen is *Chlamydia pneumonia*. Since there is a strong association between respiratory tract infections and coronary heart disease, we have a fairly simple vision of cigarette smoking increasing the disease incidence and the rate of progression by inducing repeated respiratory tract infections brought on by the pathogen that causes the disease.

We know from the days of TB that UV light has a beneficial and healing effect, Grimes said. As far as coronary heart disease is concerned, this needs to be part of a research study. Historically, TB rates were high in the British Isles; Glasgow, Scotland, in particular, was known as the tuberculosis center of Europe. More recently, it has been termed the coronary heart disease center and it has also had a particularly high incidence of osteomalacia and rickets, which are definitely the result of sunlight deficiency.

He added that it has also been found there is a much higher incidence of Crohn's disease in northwest Europe than in southern Europe. Although this is not easily explained, if we accept that Crohn's disease is also a microbial disease—probably due to *Mycobacterium paratuberculosis*—once again, sunlight in the Mediterranean area could be protective through a mechanism of immune enhancement. Multiple sclerosis is perhaps another disorder with the world's highest incidence in the northern islands of Scotland.

"The MONICA study of the World Health Organization investigated the geography of cardiovascular disease and undertook a very thorough comparison of Belfast in Northern Ireland and Toulouse in the south of France," Grimes noted. "The difference in mortality was startling. In the period of study, the number of deaths per 100,000 males, fifty-five to sixty-four years of age, in Belfast was 2,112, whereas in Toulouse it was 1,197. These are mortality rates from all causes and not just from coronary heart disease, so we must look at geography as the clue to causation."

The discussion by Grimes concerning cholesterol dovetails quite nicely with an article in the March 19, 2007, issue of *Hypertension*. Researchers at Harvard Medical School and other facilities in Boston studied 613 men and 1,198 women measuring blood levels of 25(OH)D, who were followed for four to eight years, and 38,388 men and 77,531 women with predicted vitamin D levels, who were studied for sixteen to eighteen years. An inverse association was observed between plasma 25(OH)D—25-hydroxyvitamin D—levels and risk of high blood pressure—a risk factor for heart disease.[3]

Men with vitamin D plasma levels lower than 15 ng/ml—a definite vitamin D deficiency—had more than a sixfold increase in high blood pressure compared to men with levels above 30 ng/ml. In women, those with a vitamin D deficiency showed more than a twofold increased risk for high blood pressure, compared to women with 25(OH)D levels at or above 30 ng/dl.

In studying 173 patients at high and moderate risk for coronary artery disease, vitamin D levels were inversely related to the extent of vascular calcification, according to Karol E. Watson, MD, and colleagues at the UCLA School of Medicine.[4] Their data suggests a possible role for vitamin D in the development of vascular calcification, which occurs in over 90 percent of patients with coronary heart disease.

Vitamin D is also necessary in bone mineralization, which may explain the association between osteoporosis and vascular calcification, the research team reported in *Circulation*. *Calcification* refers to the depositing of insoluble calcium salts in the body, while *vascular* relates to small blood vessels.

Among 101 patients with congestive heart failure, based on the New York

Heart Association functional class III or IV, who were candidates for transplantation, osteoporosis was present in 7 percent at the lumbar spine; 6 percent of the total hip; and 19 percent at the femoral neck, reported Elizabeth Shane, MD, and colleagues in the *American Journal of Medicine*.[5]

It was also reported that osteopenia—decreased density of bone—was reported in 43 percent at the lumbar spine, 47 percent at the total hip, and 42 percent at the femoral neck. Women were more severely affected than men.

The researchers found low levels of 25-hydroxyvitamin D and 1,25-dihydroxyvitamin D in 17 percent and 26 percent of the patients, respectively. Elevated serum parathyroid hormone levels were reported in 30 percent of the volunteers.

In addition, low blood levels of vitamin D metabolites were associated with biochemical evidence of increased bone turnover. Bone mineral density did not differ with vitamin D or parathyroid hormone status.

The researchers also reported that patients with severe congestive heart failure had significantly lower vitamin D metabolites and higher bone turnover, whereas elevated parathyroid hormone was associated with better left ventricular ejection fraction.

Since osteopenia or osteoporosis was seen in almost half the patients with severe congestive heart failure, these patients should be evaluated for vitamin D deficiency and hyperparathyroidism—that is, excessive parathyroid hormone and a disturbance in calcium metabolism, the researchers said.

A research team studied 7,186 men and 7,902 women, twenty years and older, whose data was obtained from the Third National Health and Nutrition Examination Survey. The research team evaluated the association between blood levels of 25-hydroxyvitamin D—25(OH)D—and various cardiovascular disease risk factors.[6]

The research team concluded that blood levels of vitamin D are associated with important cardiovascular disease risk factors in American adults, according to the report published in *Archives of Internal Medicine* in 2007. They added that prospective studies to assess a direct benefit of cholecalciferol—vitamin D—supplementation on cardiovascular risk factors are warranted.

As reported in the *Journal of the American College of Cardiology,* researchers studied vitamin D levels and markers of calcium metabolism in fifty-four patients with congestive heart failure. A vitamin D deficiency was common, suggesting altered calcium metabolism and abnormalities in cardiac function.[7]

According to an article published in *Acta Pediatrica,* a research team at Ulleval

Hospital in Oslo, Norway, evaluated the case of a $3^{1}/_{2}$-month old infant with severe vitamin D deficiency, hypocalcemia, hyperphosphatemia, a dilated left ventricle, severely reduced myocardial contractibility, and congestive heart failure.[8]

Calcitriol at 0.25 mcg/day was given orally from the first day in the hospital and thereafter for three weeks. Calcitriol is the second step in the biological conversion of vitamin D_3 to its active form. Treatment was then continued with cholecalciferol (vitamin D_3) at 40 mcg/day for eight weeks. The child improved remarkably, and at the time the article was written, she was three years of age and needed no medication. Although myocardial function was normal, she did have some motor delay.

The researchers are convinced that her transistory congestive heart failure was due to severe vitamin D deficiency with profound hypocalcemia (low blood levels of calcium).

As reported in the *European Heart Journal,* a forty-one-year-old woman was admitted to University Hospital of Wales in Cardiff with mild congestive heart failure that was initially controlled with diuretics (water pills), which no doubt rid the body of many essential vitamins and minerals.[9]

Her health eventually deteriorated and she had increased heart failure. She was also diagnosed with hyperphosphatemic osteomalacia, that is high phosphate levels and low vitamin D status.

Her doctor prescribed 300,000 IU of intramuscular calciferol and placed her on 500 IU of vitamin A, vitamin D, and two Sandocal supplements. Her calcium normalized and her cardiac failure improved remarkably; the research team concluded that the hypocalcemia of osteomalacia may exacerbate or even cause cardiomyopathy, and that calcium supplements may normalize the cardiac pathology.

A vitamin D deficiency is associated with a greater risk of developing cardiovascular disease for those with high blood pressure, reported Mike Mitka in the February 20, 2008, issue of the *Journal of the American Medical Association.*[10]

Thomas J. Wang, MD, and colleagues with the famous Framingham Heart Study, added that a vitamin D deficiency affects 1 billion people worldwide.

The research team followed 1,730 volunteers for an average of 5.4 years, comparing them with those without a vitamin D deficiency. This was defined as having a level of 25-dihydroxyvitamin D below 15 ng/ml.

They concluded that a deficiency of the vitamin increased the risk of developing a first cardiovascular event by 62 percent for those with a systolic (beating) pressure exceeding 139 mmHg, and a diastolic (resting) pressure exceeding 89 mmHg, or who were receiving antihypertensive therapy.

The prevalence of both high blood pressure and vitamin D insufficiency are high in the United States, according to Suzanne E. Judd et al. of Emory University School of Medicine in Atlanta, writing in the January 2008 issue of the *American Journal of Clinical Nutrition*.[11]

In fact, they continued, recent clinical and animal studies have reported that vitamin D insufficiency may be associated with elevated blood pressure, especially in Caucasians. About 30 percent of Americans are estimated to have hypertension.

In one randomized, placebo-controlled study of 145 elderly women, it was found that 400 IU of vitamin D_3, plus 600 mg of calcium daily, significantly reduced blood pressure by 9.3 percent after eight weeks, whereas treatment with 600 mg of calcium alone brought blood pressure down by only 4.0 percent.

While the cause of high blood pressure remains unknown, overweight and the dietary intake of sodium/salt, potassium, calcium, and magnesium are all aspects of nutrient intake that may have important effects on blood pressure in Americans, the research team added.

10.

Celiac Disease

Celiac disease, celiac sprue, or gluten enteropathy is a disorder in which the lining of the small intestine is damaged by gluten, a protein found in wheat, rye, oats, and barley. This damage results in malabsorption; that is, failure to absorb many important nutrients from the intestine. The patient loses weight and becomes deficient in various vitamins and minerals, according to the *American Medical Association Home Medical Encyclopedia*. This leads to anemia and a variety of skin conditions. It also results in large amounts of fat and other nutrients in the feces, resulting in bulky and foul-smelling stools.[1]

It is not clear how gluten damages the intestinal lining, the publication added. It is probably caused by an abnormal immunological response; thus, the immune system becomes sensitized to gluten and reacts to it as if it were an infection or a foreign body.

"This abnormal reaction is limited to the intestinal lining and the practical result is that the villi [frondlike projections] from the lining become flattened," the publication said. "Flattening of the villi seriously impairs their ability to absorb nutrients."

Celiac disease tends to run in families. In infants, symptoms usually occur within six months of the introduction of gluten into the diet. The feces become bulky, greasy, pale, and have an offensive odor. The baby then becomes listless and irritable, and loses weight. The baby usually produces a lot of gas and has a swollen abdomen.

Defective absorption of iron may cause iron deficiency anemia, and defective absorption of folic acid (a B vitamin) may result in megaloblastic anemia. Vomiting can lead to acute diarrhea, making the infant dehydrated and seriously ill.

Celiac disease usually develops gradually over months or years in adults, and symptoms range from vague tiredness and breathlessness—due to anemia—to weight loss, diarrhea, vomiting, abdominal pain and swelling in the legs, the publication continued. In some patients, the damage to the intestinal lining is minor, but a chronic, distinctive rash (dermatitis herpetiformis) can surface.

Doctors make a diagnosis of celiac disease with a jejunal biopsy, in which a sample of tissue is taken from the lining of the upper small intestine. It may be necessary to collect three biopsies, one when the patient is eating food containing gluten, one when the patient is on a gluten-free diet, and, finally, one when gluten is reintroduced into the diet.

"A change in the intestinal lining during the second and third biopsies indicates that the gluten is causing the illness," the publication said. "Blood, urine, and feces tests can show the extent of malabsorption."

Celiac disease is an autoimmune disease that is unique, since its environmental cause is not known, according to Peter H. R. Green, MD, of Columbia University College of Physicians and Surgeons in New York, and Christophe Cellier, MD, PhD, of the Georges Pompidou Hospital in Paris. It was originally called celiac sprue after the Dutch word *sprue,* which was used to describe a disease similar to tropical sprue that resulted in diarrhea, emaciation, aphthous stomatitis (inflammation of the mucous membranes in the mouth), and malabsorption. The disease, which occurs in both adults and children, affects about 1 percent of the population, Green and Cellier reported in the October 25, 2007, issue of the *New England Journal of Medicine.*[2]

"Although wheat, rye, and barley should be avoided . . . there are other sources of starch that can provide flours for cooking and baking," the authors said. "Since the substitute flours are not fortified with B vitamins, vitamin deficiencies may occur. This has been detected in those who have been on the diet for more than 10 years. Therefore, vitamin supplementation is advised. Meats, dairy products, and fruits and vegetables are naturally gluten free and can help to make for a more nutritious and varied diet."

Even after patients have been diagnosed with celiac disease, they should be assessed for deficiencies in vitamins and minerals, especially folic acid, vitamin B_{12}, fat-soluble vitamins (A, D, E, and K), and minerals, iron, and calcium; any such deficiencies should be treated, the authors advised. All patients should also undergo screening for osteoporosis, which has a high prevalence in this population.

"A gluten free diet fails to induce clinical or histologic improvement in 7 to 30 percent of the patients," the authors added. "Such lack of response should trigger systematic evaluation and the first step is to reassess the initial diagnosis, since villous atrophy with associated crypt hyperplasia, that is, an increase in the number of cells in a tissue or organ is not exclusive to celiac disease."

The clinical picture of celiac disease in adults includes alteration of calcium homeostatis, vitamin D levels, and bone mineral density (BMD), according to Seymour Mishkin, MD, of McGill University Health Centre in Montreal.[3]

While it is not clear to what extent treatment of celiac disease increases BMD when the treatment begins in adulthood, decreased bone mineralization is observed in untreated adults with this disorder. It is not certain whether bone mineralization is totally restored by dietary treatment started in childhood, he added.

In a study reported in the *American Journal of Gastroenterology,* Carlos Mautalen, MD, and colleagues in Buenos Aires, Argentina, evaluated fourteen patients with celiac disease. All were given a gluten-free diet. Seven were randomly selected to receive the diet only, and the other seven were randomly selected to receive a diet plus calcium at 1 g/day and vitamin D at 32,000 IU/week, given in a single dose.[4]

After one year of gluten restriction, bone mass had increased 5 percent in the lumbar spine and 5 percent in the total skeleton. In the eleven patients who adhered to the gluten-restricted diet, bone density increased 8.4 percent in the lumbar spine and 7.7 percent in the total skeleton.

Mautalen added that remineralization was more pronounced in the axial than in the peripheral skeleton. In those treated with diet only, mineralization was similar to that of patients given diet and supplements. The gluten-free diet brought a decrease in bone turnover activity, and strict gluten avoidance promoted a significant increase in bone mineral density.

Muscle wasting and hypotonia are frequently seen in the acute phase of celiac disease. Hypotonia is a reduced tension in muscles, such as in the eyeball. Muscle weakness may be a consequence of malabsorption or malnutrition with protein and/or calorie deficiency, and nutritional myopathy may develop.[5]

In chronic malabsorption, symptoms may be fatigability, limb pain or muscle cramps, hypotonia, proximal weakness due to muscular involvement secondary to vitamin D deficiency, low levels of calcium in the blood, osteomalacia, or rickets.

Disorders associated with celiac disease include autoimmune thyroid disease or rheumatoid arthritis, both of which can cause myopathy or an abnormal condition of muscular tissue, reported *Epilepsy and Other Neurological Disorders in Coeliac Disease.*

As reported in the *Journal of the American Dietetic Association,* seventeen patients with celiac disease, who had never eaten wheat starch, were compared to fourteen controls with celiac disease who tolerated wheat starch over a one-year trial for the effects of the addition of wheat starch to a gluten-free diet.[6]

Eleven of the seventeen celiac patients who had never consumed wheat starch developed symptoms, which resolved several weeks after discontinuing the product. There was a relapse of skin lesions in two of three patients with coexisting dermatitis herpetiformis.

The researchers at Hôpital Ste-Justine in Montreal suggest that long-term ingestion of gluten-free products containing wheat starch has still not been proven to be harmless. Therefore, continued use of these products in patients with celiac disease is not recommended.

At the Università di Roma in Italy, researchers evaluated a thirty-five-year-old woman with untreated celiac disease, vitamin D deficiency and subsequent hypocalcemia (low blood levels of calcium in the blood), and hyperparathyroidism, as reported the *Lancet.* Hyperparathyroidism causes an increase in the secretion of parathyroids, which causes elevated blood levels of calcium, decreased serum phosphorus, and an excretion of both minerals.[7]

The researchers found that all these conditions resulted in osteomalacia, which brings on a softening, weakening, and demineralization of bones due to a vitamin D deficiency. Healthy bones require an adequate intake of both calcium and phosphorus, but the minerals cannot be absorbed without a generous amount of vitamin D.

In reviewing available data, Jacques Schmitz, MD, of Hôpital des Enfants Malades in Paris, suggested that moderate amounts of oats, about 50 g/day or less, taken for less than a month, will probably not have an adverse effect on celiac disease. However, he reported in the *British Medical Journal,* dosages of more than 100 g/day for longer than a month will have an adverse effect on celiac disease and may aggravate the condition.[8]

Researchers at Instituto di Clinica Pediatrica in Parma, Italy, discussed two patients with celiac disease. The first was a thirty-three-year-old male who developed seizures. After being placed on a gluten-free diet for six months, anticonvulsive treatment was stopped and a biopsy found a normal gastrointestinal mucosa and the patient remained well.[9]

The second patient was a fifty-nine-year-old male with a history of diarrhea, weight loss, and depression. After being on a gluten-free diet for one month, antidepressant treatment was stopped. After one year on the gluten-free diet, he had gained weight and was in good health. A duodenal biopsy found that the intestinal mucosa was normal. The researchers said that celiac disease is probably more often misdiagnosed in adults than in children.

Whether or not oats can be safely consumed by those with celiac disease has been debated for over forty years, according to Tricia Thompson, RD. Oats are a good source of soluble fiber, and they increase the intake of the soluble fiber beta-glucan, which is found in oat bran and can possibly lower low-density lipoprotein cholesterol.[10] However, definitive dietary recommendations regarding the place of oats in the gluten-free diet cannot be made on the basis of current research, Thompson said.

As reported in the *American Journal of Clinical Nutrition,* bone mineral content of 33 celiac patients was found to be significantly lower than in 225 controls. In 14 patients, the bone mineral content increased significantly after 1.28 years of a gluten-free diet.[11]

The researchers at Clinica Pediatrica III in Milan, Italy, concluded that osteoporosis complicates celiac disease during childhood and adolescence and that a gluten-free diet alone is able to markedly improve bone mineralization.

In the United Kingdom, the prevalence of celiac disease is about 1 in 200, and the disease peaks in childhood between two and three years of age, according to Peter Howdle, MD, of St. James University Hospital in Leeds, United Kingdom.[12]

It is common for celiac disease patients to develop gastrointestinal symptoms or symptoms of nutritional deficiency. Weight loss, diarrhea, and fatigue often occur. On occasion, rickets from a vitamin D deficiency or bleeding from a vitamin K deficiency is common.

Other causes of small bowel abnormalities in the intestinal mucosa include cow's milk protein intolerance, soy protein intolerance, immunodeficiency syndrome, eosinophile gastroenteropathy, intractable diarrhea of infancy, gastroenteritis in children, parasites, tuberculosis, HIV, contaminated bowel syndrome, Whipple's disease (a bacterial infection), tropical sprue, arterial disease of the small intestine, and drug and radiation damage, Howdle said.

Fundamentals of the Gluten-free Diet

Grains That Should Be Avoided: Wheat (spelt, kamut, semolina, triticale), rye, barley (including malt)

Safe Grains (Gluten-free): Rice, amaranth, buckwheat, corn, millet, quinoa, sorghum, teff (an Ethiopian cereal grain), and oats*

Gluten-Free Starches That Can Be Used for Flour Alternatives: Cereal grains, amaranth, buckwheat, corn (polenta), millet, quinoa, sorghum, teff, rice (white, brown, wild, basmati, jasmine), montina (Indian rice grass)

Tubers: Arrowroot, jicama, taro, potato, tapioca (cassava, manioc, yucca)

Legumes: Chickpeas, lentils, kidney beans, navy beans, peas, peanuts, soybeans

Nuts: Almonds, walnuts, chestnuts, hazelnuts, cashews

Seeds: Sunflower, flax, pumpkin

---

*Clinical studies suggest that oats are tolerated by most patients with celiac disease and may improve the nutritional content of the diet. However, oats are not uniformly recommended because most commercially available oats are contaminated with gluten-containing grains during the growing, transportation, and milling processes.

Source: Green and Cellier, "Celiac Disease." See note 2, this chapter.

1 1 .

Crohn's Disease

Named after Burrill Crohn, an American gastroenterologist (1884–1983), Crohn's disease is a chronic inflammation that can affect any part of the gastrointestinal tract, ranging from the mouth to the anus. It can cause pain, fever, diarrhea, and weight loss, according to the *American Medical Association Home Medical Guide.*[1]

The most common site of inflammation is the terminal ileum—the end of the small intestine where it joins the large intestine. In this disorder, the intestinal wall becomes very thick, due to chronic inflammation, and develops deep, penetrating ulcers. The condition tends to be patchy, in that areas of the intestine that lie between diseased areas may appear normal, but they are usually mildly affected.

"The cause of Crohn's disease is unknown, but it may represent an abnormal allergic reaction or it may be an exaggerated response to an infectious agent, such as a bacterium or a virus," the publication said. "There is a slight genetic predisposition or inherited tendency to develop the disease. A person may be affected at any age, but the peak ages are in adolescence and early adulthood and after 60."

In young people, the ileum is usually involved, and the disease causes spasms of pain in the abdomen, diarrhea, and chronic sickness due to loss of appetite, anemia, and weight loss. The ability of the small intestine to absorb food is impaired.

In the elderly, it is more common for the disease to affect the rectum, causing rectal bleeding, the publication added. The disease may also affect the anus, causing chronic abscesses, deep cracks, and fistulas (passageways that create an abnormal link between organs of the body).

"Crohn's disease can also affect the colon (large intestine), causing bloody diarrhea," the publication continued. "It is rare in the mouth, esophagus, stomach, and duodenum (upper part of the small intestine). Complications may affect the intestines or they may develop elsewhere in the body. Thickening of the intestinal wall may narrow the inside diameter so much that an intestinal obstruction develops."

It is estimated that 30 percent of patients with this disease develop a fistula. Internal fistulas may form between loops of the intestine. External fistulas on the skin of the abdomen or the skin surrounding the anus may follow a surgical operation or rupture of an abscess. This can cause leakage of feces through the skin.

Abscesses (pus-filled pockets of infection) form in about 20 percent of patients with Crohn's disease, which is also called regional enteritis. These pockets can occur around the anus or within the abdomen.

Complications in other parts of the body may include inflammation of the eye, severe arthritis affecting various joints of the body, ankylosing spondylitis (inflammation of the spine), and skin disorders such as eczema, the publication said.

A sigmoidoscopy, an examination of the rectum with a viewing tube, may confirm presence of the disease in the rectum. X-rays using barium meals or barium enemas will show thickened loops of bowel with deep fissures. It is often difficult to distinguish between Crohn's disease, which affects the colon, and ulcerative colitis, which is limited to the large intestine. A colonoscopy, an examination of the colon using a flexible viewing tube, or biopsy (the removal of tissue for microscopic examination), may help to determine which disorder is present. Blood tests often show evidence of protein deficiency or anemia.

Severe acute attacks may require a hospital stay for blood transfusions, intravenous feeding, and drug therapy, the publication added. The severity of the disease fluctuates widely, and the patient is often under long-term medical care. Some patients find that certain foods exacerbate their symptoms. Others may benefit from a high-vitamin, low-fiber diet.

A surgical procedure to remove damaged portions of the intestine may be necessary to treat chronic obstruction or blood loss. If the small intestine is involved, the surgeon may remove the most affected parts, although surgery is not a cure-all. If the large intestine is affected, surgery may involve removal of narrowed obstructing segments, the publication said.

According to an article in *Gastroenterology,* researchers evaluated forty normal volunteers and eighty-two patients with Crohn's disease and found that 65 percent of those with Crohn's disease had low blood levels of 25-hydroxyvita-min D; in 25 percent there were deficient levels of the vitamin.[2]

In addition, those who had the lowest 25-hydroxyvitamin D levels were those with previous ileal reactions. In a subgroup of nine patients, six had osteomalacia and three had osteoporosis. After nine and eighteen months of oral vitamin D at 4,000 IU/day (0.1 mg), three of those with osteomalacia and low vitamin D levels showed histologic improvement after the oral vitamin D supplementation normalized blood levels of 25-hydroxyvitamin D. Osteomalacia is the gradual softening of bone. The softening develops because the bones contain osteoid tissue that fails to calcify due to a lack of vitamin D.

In three patients with metabolic bone disease who had normal blood levels of vitamin D at the time of diagnosis there was no histologic improvement following vitamin D therapy, the researchers said.

In a study involving thirty-one men and forty-four women between the ages of sixteen and seventy-seven who had Crohn's disease, participants were randomly assigned to receive either oral vitamin D at 1,000 IU/day for one year or no supplement. In 57 percent of the patients who were given the supplement, blood levels of 25-hydroxyvitamin D increased, compared with 37 percent in the controls.[3]

The researchers, reporting in the *European Journal of Gastroenterology and Hepatology*, said that bone mineral density decreased significantly in the nonsupplemented group, but not in those given vitamin D.

In those who received vitamin D and had normal blood levels of 25-hydroxyvitamin D, 68 percent had increases in bone mineral density when compared with 18 percent of the volunteers with low blood levels of the vitamin. Those who did not have an intestinal resection and were given the vitamin had slightly greater increases in bone mineral density than those who had undergone intestinal resection or surgery.

In twelve patients with Crohn's disease and intestinal resections and four normal controls, absorption of cholecalciferol and 25-hydroxycholecalciferol was reduced in those with Crohn's disease to the extent of the resection of the small bowel, reported the *American Journal of Clinical Nutrition*. Cholecalciferol is vitamin D_3; 25-hydroxycholecalciferol is the initial step in the biological conversion of vitamin D_3 to the more active form—calcidiol—which is more potent than vitamin D_3 (also called calcifediol).[4]

The researchers found that 25-hydroxycholecalciferol absorption was greater than that of cholecalciferol (vitamin D_3). Vitamin D malabsorption that occurs in patients with Crohn's disease is due to the extent of distal small bowel resection. In those with severe short bowel syndrome, 25-hydroxycholecalciferol supplements may be necessary, while in those with small or moderate resections, oral cholecalciferol may be sufficient.

A resection is the surgical removal of part or all of a diseased or injured organ or structure. If the patient does not respond to medical treatment, surgical removal of part of the intestine may be necessary. However, since the disease may recur even after surgical removal of the abnormality, medical treatment is often used whenever possible before surgery is considered.[5]

According to an article in *Gut,* researchers evaluated eighteen men and twenty-two women, ranging in age from eighteen to sixty-eight, who had Crohn's disease. It was found that blood levels of 25-hydroxycholecalciferol were reduced in the undernourished Crohn's disease patients when compared to those with the disease who were well nourished.[6]

Over 50 percent of the undernourished Crohn's disease patients had evidence of secondary hyperparathyroidism and elevated alkaline phosphatase levels. Hyperparathyroidism causes an increase in the secretion of parathyroids, which results in elevated blood levels of calcium, decreased blood levels of phosphorus, and an increased excretion of calcium and phosphorus.

The researchers added that low levels of 25-hydroxycholecalciferol were related to disease activity and that undernourished patients with Crohn's disease who have high levels of the disease are at risk for vitamin D deficiency and are in need of supplementation.

Exposure to sunlight in these patients may be of benefit during the winter months, the researchers added. Avoidance of drugs such as cholestyramine, which can lower 25-hydroxycholecalciferol levels, is recommended. Cholestyramine is a drug that binds dietary cholesterol and prevents its absorption.

Inflammatory bowel disease (IBD) patients have an increased risk of diminished vitamin and mineral status for a number of reasons, including anorexia, restrictive diets, malabsorption due to disease or surgery, diarrhea, bleeding of the intestinal mucosa, or drug-nutrient interactions, as reported in *Family Practice News.*[7]

Among Crohn's disease patients, low vitamin B_{12} levels range from 5 percent to 60 percent; low levels of folic acid (a B vitamin) are 3–64 percent; and in vitamin D, low levels range from 25 percent to 65 percent among IBD patients. All IBD patients are prone to low blood levels of folic acid, and when these levels drop more than 5 ng/ml, blood homocysteine rises, increasing the risk of atherosclerotic vascular disease.

Prednisone and cholestyramine, which are frequently used in IBD, inhibit the action of vitamin D, the publication said. Vitamin D levels also drop, depending on the season. One researcher has recommended supplementing IBD patients with one to two times the recommended daily allowance of vitamin D of 200 to 400 IU/day.

Although iron deficiency is common among these patients, oral supplementation with the mineral may not be recommended since it may cause nausea and vomiting. However, if the deficiency is more than 300 mg, parenteral supplementation (that is, by injection) may be necessary.

Although food allergy has long been considered an important causative factor in the development of IBD, it is only recently that there have been studies utilizing a diet that eliminates foods that cause allergies in the treatment of Crohn's disease and ulcerative colitis, according to Michael T. Murray, ND.[8]

For example, in a controlled trial of twenty patients with Crohn's disease, ten patients were put on a diet that excluded allergy-causing foods and the other ten were given a high-fiber diet. At the end of six months, seven out of the ten on the allergy-elimination diet remained symptom-free, compared with none of the ten in the other group.

"In another study of patients with Crohn's disease, the allergy eliminating diet allowed fifty-one out of seventy-seven patients to remain on the diet alone without medications for periods up to fifty-one months," Murray added. "Since Crohn's disease and ulcerative colitis are currently treated with corticosteroids, harsh drugs that impair the immune system, and, since surgery is most often ineffective and produces numerous undesirable side effects, the results of these studies suggest that elimination of allergy causing foods should be considered as treatment for Crohn's disease and ulcerative colitis."

A seventy-one-year-old woman was admitted to the hospital because of left-sided weakness and a mass in the brain, reported Daniel K. Podolsky, MD, and colleagues at the Massachusetts General Hospital in Boston and other facilities. The patient had had Crohn's disease for many years, but she was in her usual state of health until three months before admission, when she became fatigued and required daily naps. Two months prior to admission, episodes of blurred vision, occipital headaches, and an unsteady gait occurred.[9]

Two weeks before admission, the patient noted an enlarging, nontender mass in her right inguinal (groin) area. Later, nausea developed, the patient's appetite decreased, and, over the course of the next week, she lost weight.

A team of specialists reviewed the patient's history and reported that it has long been suspected there is an increased frequency of lymphoma in cases of Crohn's disease, although this premise remains controversial. They added that the patient has at least three possible risk factors for non-Hodgkin's lymphoma—Crohn's disease, immunosuppressive therapy with mercaptopurine (an antiplastic agent), and infliximab therapy. While the impact of each risk factor alone may be small, the overall effect may be additive, if not synergistic, said Podolsky.

He added, "Accordingly, I believe that lymphoma may have developed in the patient, probably large B-cell lymphoma that is positive for the Epstein-Barr virus."

Although the doctors did not discuss the causes of lymphoma—or nutritional overtones—I have decided to include this case history in the event that it may shed new light on the development of Crohn's disease.

Non-Hodgkin's lymphoma is any cancer of lymphoid tissue that is found mainly in the lymph nodes and spleen, other than Hodgkin's disease. These cancers vary in their malignancy according to the nature and activity of the abnormal cells.[10]

While the cause of non-Hodgkin's lymphoma is not known, the disease is sometimes associated with the suppression of the immune system (see studies noted below). One type of non-Hodgkin's lymphoma, called Burkitt's lymphoma, is thought to be caused by the Epstein-Barr virus.

1. In a study of 35,000 Iowa women, aged fifty-five to sixty-nine, 104 cases of non-Hodgkin's lymphoma were recorded. Relative risk of the disease was related to saturated and monounsaturated fat (Brian Chiu et al., "Diet and Risk of Non-Hodgkin's Lymphoma in Older Women," *JAMA* 275, no. 17 [1996]: 1315–1321).

2. In 156 cases of non-Hodgkin's lymphoma, compared to 527 controls, consumption of community water with high levels of nitrates was a risk factor. Those with lower intakes of vitamin C were at a slightly higher risk (Mary H. Ward et al., "Drinking Water Nitrates and the Risk of Non-Hodgkin's Lymphoma," *Epidemiology* 7, no. 5 [September 1996]: 465–471).

3. Lack of sunlight exposure is a risk factor. This disease is significantly lower in the southern half of the United States—because of vitamin D availability—

according to a survey from 1950 to 1980 (Patricia Hartge, ScD, "Non-Hodgkin's Lymphoma and Sunlight," *Journal of the National Cancer Institute* 88, no. 5 [March 6, 1996]: 298–300).

4. Exposure to pesticides and other agricultural chemicals are risk factors for non-Hodgkin's lymphoma (K. P. Cantor et al, "Pesticides and Other Agricultural Risk Factors for Non-Hodgkin's Lymphoma among Men in Iowa and Minnesota," *Cancer Research* 52 [May 1, 1992]: 2447–2455).

5. In evaluating 268 children who developed non-Hodgkin's lymphoma, there was an increased risk for those exposed to pesticides in the home and from professional exterminations in the home (J. D. Buckley et al., "Pesticide Exposure in Children with Non-Hodgkin's Lymphoma," *Cancer* 89, no. 1 [December 1, 2000]: 2315–2321).

6. Exposure to PCBs and organochlorines may be immunotoxic and increase the risk for non-Hodgkin's lymphoma (Lennart Hardell et al., "Polychlorinated Biphenyls, Chlordanes, and the Etiology of Non-Hodgkin's Lymphoma," *Epidemiology* 8, no. 6 [November 1997]: 689).

7. Exposure to solvents and meatpacking processing increased the risk of non-Hodgkin's lymphoma (Lilith Tathum, "Risk Factors for Subgroups of Non-Hodgkin's Lymphoma," *Epidemiology* 8, no. 5 [1997]: 551–558).

1 2.

Cystic Fibrosis

When cystic fibrosis (CF) was initially identified in the 1930s, before effective antibiotics were available, almost all CF patients died in early childhood, explained the *American Medical Association Home Medical Encyclopedia*. Since 1975, the outlook has changed dramatically, especially with advanced methods of diagnosis and treatment.[1]

CF, or mucoviscidosis, is caused by a defective gene. This defect is of the recessive type, suggesting that it must be inherited in a double dose (one gene from each parent). Those who inherit the defective gene from one parent are called carriers, and they are usually unaware they have the disease and have no symptoms.

With CF, certain glands do not function properly, especially the glands in the lining of the bronchial tubes, the publication said. An additional serious malfunction is the failure of the pancreas to produce enzymes involved in the breakdown of fats and their absorption from the intestines, thus causing malnutrition. Sweat glands are also affected.

"To enable food to be properly digested, replacement pancreatic enzyme must be taken with meals," the publication continued. "The diet needs to be rich in calories and proteins and a vitamin supplement is often prescribed as an extra precaution. These measures bring about weight increase and more normal feces."

Low bone mineral density has been well-documented in people with cystic fibrosis, and while bone disease in this disorder is likely complicated, a vitamin D deficiency has been implicated as a causative factor, according to Anne Stephenson and colleagues at St. Michael's Hospital in Toronto, and colleagues at other facilities.[2]

They pointed out that vitamin D is essential in maintaining bone health, since it maximizes calcium absorption from the lumen (the cavity of an organ) of the gut. A 25-hydroxyvitamin D (25(OH)D) deficiency has been found in CF patients in spite of routine supplementation.

Typically, a blood level 25(OH)D of less than 20 ng/ml is considered a deficiency; however, more recent research has suggested that more of the vitamin is perhaps needed.

The reasons for a vitamin D deficiency in CF patients include: (1) decreased gastrointestinal absorption; (2) impaired hydroxylation of vitamin D; (3) reduced sun exposure; (4) increased use of sunscreen; (5) seasonal influences; and (6) geographical location.

"Several forms of vitamin D supplementation have been used to correct vitamin D deficiency; however, controversy exists as to the most effective way of administering vitamin D to cystic fibrosis patients," the researchers added. "Hanly, et al., assessed the response to 800 IU/day of vitamin D_3 (cholecalciferol) in 20 adolescents and young adults with CF and found that blood concentrations of 25(OH)D increased from 10.3 to 21.3 nmol/l, although concentrations in many of the patients remained well below the target range" (J. G. Hanly et al., *Quarterly Journal of Medicine* 56 [1985]: 377–385).

The Canadian study involved 360 adults with CF; 249 of them (69 percent) had 25(OH)D concentrations at the beginning of the study of less than 20 ng/ml, in spite of similar levels of supplementation. The lowest concentrations of the vitamin were found in younger patients, who had lower body mass indexes and less lung function. However, vitamin D concentrations increased significantly in 92 percent of the patients following intervention.

Intervention involved oral intake of cholecalciferol in one of two ways: either the patient was counseled on compliance or additional oral cholecalciferol was added to the patient's regimen. If the concentration was 20 ng/ml, the dietitian contacted the patient, reviewed the dosage the patient was taking, and inquired about compliance. For those who were not following orders, the dietitian encouraged compliance and reviewed the importance of adequate vitamin D supplementation, reminding them of the impact on their health.

"If the patient was compliant with the regimen, additional oral calciferol was prescribed with increases as follows: 17 percent added 400 IU/day; 5 percent added 800 IU/day; 61 percent added 1,000 IU/day; and 17 percent added more than 1,000 IU/day," the researchers said.

The research team concluded that vitamin D concentrations of less than 20 ng/ml are common in CF patients. And bringing low amounts within the normal range may mitigate the deleterious effects of chronic vitamin D deficiency. Although the most effective way to normalize concentrations is unknown, the 2005 CFF Consensus Statement on bone health recommends supplementation with high-dose ergocalciferol (D_2).

"Our data imply that young CF patients with low lung function and a low body mass index may be at the highest risk of vitamin D deficiency and should be monitored closely," the researchers said. "Sun exposure may be required to achieve higher concentrations in CF patients; however, further studies are needed to evaluate the use of UV light exposure to maximize vitamin D synthesis in the skin."

At St. James University Hospital, Leeds, United Kingdom, Rosemary J. Rayner reviewed the importance of fat-soluble vitamins (A, D, E, and K) in CF patients. Since these patients have other serious medical problems, nutritional evaluation may often be overlooked.[3]

Pancreatic insufficiency at birth can result in fat malabsorption of the four vitamins; however, pancreatic enzyme replacement therapy and routine vitamin supplementation can eliminate many clinical deficiencies of these vitamins in children who are diagnosed and treated early, she said.

She goes on to say that CF patients are still at risk for vitamin deficiency if the diagnosis is made late, if part of the bowel has been resected (partially removed), or if fat-soluble vitamin supplements are not taken. CF patients are known to be deficient in these vitamins.

Sample dosages of vitamins A, D, and E in CF children or adults are: 2.4 mg/day of vitamin A; 20 mcg/day of vitamin D; and 100 to 200 IU/day of vitamin E. As the prognosis for CF patients continues to improve, clinical problems due to fat-soluble vitamin deficiencies will become more prevalent. Those at risk are patients with severe malabsorption, poor compliance, or those with liver disease, Rayner added.

There is considerable evidence that fat-soluble vitamins are at the lowest end of the normal spectrum in patients with cystic fibrosis, in spite of supplementation, according to Siobhan Carr, MD, and colleagues. Therefore, a tailored approach aimed at pushing each patient's vitamin needs into the higher end of the normal range may be necessary.[4] The researchers drew the following conclusions:

- Vitamin A is important for immune function and respiratory epithelium integrity. Beta-carotene (provitamin A) is beneficial for antioxidant defenses.

Recommended intake of vitamin A in infants is roughly 5,000 IU/day; in two- to eight-year-olds, 5,000 IU/day; and in those over eight, 5,000–10,000 IU/day.

- Vitamin D is important in bone metabolism. Recommended vitamin D supplementation in CF children between birth and eight years of age is 400 IU/day and for those over eight, 800 IU/day.

- Vitamin E is necessary in antioxidant defenses. Recommended vitamin E supplementation in CF infants is between 25 and 100 IU/day; for those two to eight years old, between 100 and 200 IU/day; and for those ten and older, 200–400 IU/day.

- Vitamin K is important in coagulation (blood clotting) and bone metabolism. Recommended vitamin K supplementation in CF patients less than one year old should be 2.5 mg/week; those over one, between 5 and 10 mg/week.

- Vitamin C, which is water-soluble, is important in antioxidant defense. Recommended vitamin C supplementation should be between 30 and 60 mg/day.

In studying 54 patients with cystic fibrosis, ranging in age from 4.9 to 19.5 years, compared with 160 other pediatric patients living in the same region, there were low-normal levels of 25-hydroxyvitamin D and a high prevalence of low (18 percent) and marginal (18 percent) levels of 1,25-dihydroxyvitamin D, according to an article published in the *Southern Medical Journal*.[5]

The researchers added that malabsorption and inadequate supplementation did not account for the finding and the cause was uncertain.

Cystic fibrosis is a multisystem disease, characterized primarily by chronic pulmonary infection and bronchiectasis (dilation of bronchi), pancreatic exocrine impairment (*exocrine* refers to a gland that excretes outwardly), and elevated sweat chloride, according to Michael P. Boyle, MD, of the Johns Hopkins University School of Medicine in Baltimore.[6]

However, he continued, in the past forty years, new treatment strategies and aggressive nutritional management have resulted in a significant increase in life expectancy, with a median predicted survival in CF now higher than thirty-five years.

He added that it is estimated that within the next decade more than half of all individuals with CF will be eighteen or older, and adult medicine caregivers are increasingly likely to encounter patients with CF and be called on to manage their illness.

Writing in the October 17, 2007, issue of the *Journal of the American Medical Association,* Boyle discussed a fifty-two-year-old man with CF and the protocol the author recommended for dealing with the disease. In his twenties and thirties, the patient was very active and his health care consisted of occasionally seeing an internist, taking pancreatic enzymes, and inhaling albuterol when needed. By his forties, however, he began to have worsening shortness of breath and more frequent lung infections. He also developed severe sinusitis, which required surgery.

In studying CF patients, Boyle said that by the time they reach adulthood, 20–30 percent develop pancreatic endocrine insufficiency, in addition to their exocrine insufficiency. CF-related diabetes is a unique form of the disease that has characteristics different from both type 1 and type 2 diabetes, in that the pancreas produces a small amount of insulin, but in insufficient quantities to metabolize carbohydrates.

This condition almost never results in ketoacidosis—large amounts of glucose in the blood—but it is frequently characterized by significant hyperglycemia (high amounts of glucose in the blood) following a meal.

"Poorly controlled diabetes, which can result in neutrophil (white blood cells) dysfunction and malnutrition, is associated with accelerated loss of lung function and increased mortality in those with CF," Boyle continued. "Other common endocrine complications of adult CF include osteopenia (decreased density of bone) and osteoporosis (atrophy of skeletal tissue), with about two thirds of adults with CF demonstrating decreased bone mineral content."

While vitamin D deficiency is extremely common in adults with CF and often contributes to decreased bone density, the decreased bone mineral content seen in CF is likely the result of multiple factors, including chronic inflammatory cytokines, inadequate testosterone levels, malnutrition, and direct effect of CFTR mutations on bone development, he said. Cytokines are hormonelike proteins that regulate the intensity of immune responses. CFTR is a protein involved in sodium and water balance.

Boyle goes on to say that 90 percent of CF patients have pancreatic exocrine insufficiency, which requires them to take oral pancreatic enzyme supplements with meals to prevent chronic malabsorption. These supplements generally contain a mixture of enzymes that catalyze the hydrolysis of starch, proteins, and fats, such as amylase, lipase, and protease.

Even with these supplements, CF patients experience a degree of fat malabsorption, Boyle continued. The combination of fat malabsorption and chronic pulmonary disease often results in extremely high caloric requirements. This necessitates eating high-calorie meals, along with high-salt meals to counterbalance excess sweat sodium loss. The patient also needs extra amounts of vitamins A, D, E, and K.

Alisha J. Rovnar and colleagues at Children's Hospital in Philadelphia and the University of Pennsylvania found a vitamin D insufficiency in most of the children, adolescents, and young adults with CF in all seasons, in spite of vitamin D supplementation.[7]

Future studies should focus on identifying the optimal dose needed to maintain 25(OH)D levels between 30 and 60 ng/dl. Since CF patients are prone to osteopenia and osteoporosis, attention should be given to maintaining adequate vitamin D levels, they added.

13.

Díabetes

According to the American Diabetes Association, the grim statistics about the growing incidence of diabetes around the world indicate a widening epidemic.[1] Consider the following:

United States

- 20.8 million Americans have diabetes.

- 6.2 million Americans are unaware they have diabetes.

- 54 million Americans have prediabetes, which can quickly spread to full-blown diabetes.

- Every 21 seconds, someone in the United States is diagnosed with diabetes.

India

- Has the highest number of people with diabetes in the world—40.9 million.

China

- 64.3 million Chinese have impaired glucose tolerance, the most in the world.

Mexico

- Diabetes is responsible for 20.2 percent of all deaths.

Nauru

- This Micronesian island nation has the world's highest rate of diabetes in the adult population: 30.7 percent.

Australia

- Obesity rates in children increased by as much as four times between 1985 and 1997.

Brazil

- 50.9 percent of the people with type 2 diabetes have diabetic neuropathy. This is a disease of the nervous system or a form of nerve damage.

Finland

- Has the highest incidence rate for type 1 diabetes in children—up to the age of 14—in the world.

Europe

- Because of the region's large percentage of people over age 50, nearly 10 percent are expected to have diabetes by 2025.

United Arab Emirates

- Second-highest rate of diabetes in the adult population in the world: 19.5 percent.

Mozambique

- Residents requiring insulin will, on average, die within twelve months.

Diabetes mellitus is a disorder in which the pancreas does not produce enough insulin, the hormone responsible for the absorption of glucose (sugar) into cells for their energy needs and into the liver and fat cells for storage for later use, if needed, reported the *American Medical Association Home Medical Encyclopedia.*[2]

As a consequence, the level of glucose in the blood becomes abnormally high, which causes excessive urination and constant thirst and hunger. Since the body cannot store or use glucose properly, this causes weight loss and fatigue. Diabetes also causes a disordered lipid (fat) metabolism and accelerated degeneration of small blood vessels.

There are two main types of diabetes. Type 1 (insulin-dependent), the more severe form commonly appears in people under the age of thirty-five and especially between the ages of ten and sixteen. It develops rapidly when the insulin-secreting cells in the pancreas are destroyed, often by an immune response following a viral infection. Insulin production ceases immediately, and without insulin injections, the patient may die.

Type 2 diabetes (noninsulin-dependent) develops gradually and it is discovered only during a routine medical examination. The body produces a small amount of insulin, but it is usually not enough to meet the body's needs, especially when the person is overweight. While this type of diabetes usually develops in those over forty, type 2 is increasingly found in children because of their obesity.

A third type of diabetes is gestational diabetes, which develops in women during their third trimester of pregnancy. The disease may or may not abate after the baby is born. But if patients with gestational diabetes remain obese, the disease can reappear.

The body is often resistant to the effects of insulin (a condition known as insulin resistance), but in most cases, insulin-replacement injections are not required, since dietary measures, weight reduction, and oral medications usually keep the condition under control.

"Although obesity is the primary cause of unmasking latent diabetes, other causes can unmask or aggravate diabetes and certain illnesses, such as pancreatitis and thyrotoxicosis; certain drugs (corticosteroids and some diuretics [water pills]); infections; and, of course, pregnancy," the publication added.

With type 2 diabetes on the rise and sobering predictions for future adverse health effects as a result, experts are trying to find ways to slow the growing incidence of the disease, reported Tracy Hampton, PhD, in the August 8, 2007, issue of the *Journal of the American Medical Association.* While prevention efforts have proved difficult, researchers have discovered that significant strides can be made through programs that encourage lifestyle changes.[3]

Hampton went on to say that encouraging findings have been reported by an intervention project in North Carolina, which was discussed at the American Diabetes Association's 67th Scientific Sessions, held in June 2007 in Chicago. The project involved implementing community-based health promotion, outreach, and diabetes care incentives in Raleigh—specifically diabetes management and nutrition courses, organized walking programs, and diabetes screenings.

Diabetes rates were then tracked over an eight-year period and compared with those of a control community eighty miles (129km) away—Greensboro—that has similar demographics.

During the trial period, rates of obesity did not change in the two communities, but among individuals with body mass indexes of more than 30, there were significantly fewer cases of diabetes in the Raleigh contingent, as compared with those in Greensboro, Hampton continued.

Since the researchers found statistically significant changes in healthy behavior, weight management behavior, and diabetes prevalence in the North Carolina communities, Desmond Williams, MD, PhD, the project manager, said that "We think project DIRECT [Diabetes Intervention Reaching and Educating Communities Together] can serve as a model for other community based diabetes prevention projects."

Hampton also discussed the Finnish Diabetes Prevention Study, which involved five hundred middle-aged, overweight people with impaired glucose tolerance, in which cumulative incidence of diabetes after four years was 11 percent in the intervention group—which included individualized counseling aimed at reducing weight and fat intake and increasing physical activity, along with fiber intake—compared with 23 percent in the controls. Overall, there was a 58 percent reduction in the risk of diabetes in the intervention group.

During the follow-up period, the incidence of type 2 diabetes was 4.3 and 7.4 per one hundred person-years in the intervention and control groups, respectively, which indicated a 43 percent reduction in relative risk of diabetes in the intervention group.

The impact of the menopause transition on osteoporosis in type 1 diabetes is not well-established, according to Elsa S. Strotmeyer, PhD, and colleagues at the University of Pittsburgh in Pennsylvania. They reported that the Nord-Trodelag Health Survey and the Iowa Women's Health Survey found a seven- to twelvefold increase in hip fractures, respectively, in older type 1 diabetic women.[4]

Type 1 diabetes was associated with about a 10 percent lower bone mineral density when those with type 1 diabetes were compared with nondiabetic women in most, but not all, studies. However, many of the studies included only small numbers of patients and did not adjust for traditional osteoporosis risks, such as lower body weight and smoking.

The researchers added that genetic variants in the vitamin D receptor or collagen type 1-alpha-1 are positively associated with low bone mineral density in type 1 diabetics.

"Type 1 diabetic women with lower bone mineral density before menopause may be at an even greater risk for osteoporosis and osteopenia after the

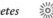

menopausal transition compared with non-diabetic women," the researchers said. "Type 1 diabetic women may experience an earlier decrease in bone mineral density due to aging, given their younger age at menopause. Since our data and several recent studies indicate that type 1 diabetic women are at a markedly increased risk for fractures, osteoporosis screening or fracture prevention efforts may be appropriate for women with type 1 diabetes."

The researchers evaluated bone mineral density and diabetes as independent variables, while adjusting for age, total lean and fat mass, height, waist-to-hip ratio, current smoking and drinking habits, exercise, menstrual cycle length, current hormone use, education, self-reported health problems, thyroid-stimulating-hormone level, hemoglobin A1C, blood pressure, diabetic-related complications (neuropathy, retinopathy, etc.), osteoporosis medications (calcitonin, fluoride, etc.), calcium and vitamin D supplement use, thiazide diuretic use, and statin use.

Osteopenia is decreased calcification or density of bone, while osteoporosis is a reduction in the quantity of bone or atrophy of skeletal tissue. The connection between calcium and vitamin D and these conditions is explored in greater detail elsewhere in this book.

According to a number of studies, circulating amounts of vitamin D may be inversely related to the prevalence of diabetes, to the concentration of glucose, and to insulin resistance, reported researchers at the Centers for Disease Control and Prevention (CDC) in Atlanta. Also, a vitamin D deficiency may be related to the metabolic syndrome—formerly called Syndrome X, an array of health conditions related to diabetes. These include high blood pressure, impaired glucose regulation, obesity, and high levels of cholesterol and triglycerides. Anyone with three of the five conditions may be a candidate for diabetes.[5]

"Because of the close interrelationships between vitamin D, parathyroid hormone, calcium, and phosphate, untangling the contributions of each of these factors on insulin resistance and glucose homeostasis (balance) is important in developing possible future approaches in the prevention of insulin resistance, the metabolic syndrome, and diabetes," said Earl S. Ford, MD, MPH, the lead researcher.

A number of clinical studies report that low 25-hydroxyvitamin D_3 concentrations may be inversely associated with type 2 diabetes, metabolic syndrome, insulin resistance, and cardiovascular disease, according to Massimo Cigolini, MD, and colleagues at the Hospital of Arzignano in Venice, Italy. Since C-reactive protein and fibrinogen levels increase the risk for cardiovascular disease (CVD), these findings could help explain the increase in CVD typically observed during winter months, a period in which vitamin D status tends to be poor and suggests a rationale for vitamin D supplementation in the prevention of CVD, especially among the elderly, Cigolini added.[6]

"Low vitamin D_3 concentrations result in elevations of parathyroid hormone, which has been linked to insulin resistance and significant increase in the serum levels of many acute phase proteins," Cigolini said. "Evidently, these findings are all consistent with the proposition that hypovitaminosis D and subsequent secondary hyperparathyroidism may promote the acute phase response and may help to explain how hypovitaminosis D might act as a risk factor for CVD."

As reported in *Diabetes Care,* David J. Di Cesar, MD, and colleagues at the State University of New York and the Department of Veterans Affairs Medical Center in Syracuse, stated that their findings suggest that vitamin D deficiency is more common in type 2 diabetes than in type 1 diabetes, unrelated to age, sex, or insulin treatment.[7]

"Despite most type 2 diabetics being prescribed a daily multivitamin, usually containing 400 IU of vitamin D, the percent who were deficient remained unchanged," Di Cesar said. "Further studies are needed to better understand the causes and clinical significance of the observed hypovitaminosis D and to investigate response to vitamin D replacement therapy."

In evaluating 238 newly diagnosed patients with impaired glucose tolerance, blood levels of vitamin D were significantly lower in the diabetics than in those with impaired glucose tolerance, as reported in an article published in *Diabetes Research and Clinical Practice.*[8]

A research team in Sweden found that vitamin D supplementation was associated with a reduced risk of type 1 diabetes. They added that most European studies indicate that vitamin D supplementation has a positive effect on infants. They theorize that the vitamin may contribute to immune modulation and protect against or arrest an ongoing immune process begun in susceptible children by early environmental exposures.[9]

As reported in *Diabetologia,* 142 elderly Dutchmen ranging in age from seventy to eighty-eight were evaluated for their vitamin D status. It was found that 39 percent were deficient in the vitamin. A one-hour glucose test and area under the glucose curve were inversely associated with blood concentrations of 25-hydroxyvitamin D. With the exclusion of newly diagnosed diabetics, total insulin concentrations during the glucose test were inversely associated with the concentrations of vitamin D.[10]

In an article in *Diabetes and Nutrition Metabolism,* a research team reported that viruses are potential inducers of beta-cell damage and that a number of viruses have reportedly been associated with type 1 diabetes, such as the enteroviruses. Other viruses that may be involved with diabetes include mumps, measles, cytomegalo (which causes cellular enlargement), and retroviruses. Beta cells in the pancreas in the Islets of Langerhans make and release insulin.[11]

A vitamin D deficiency may contribute to type 1 diabetes in childhood, the researchers added. Other factors in the disease may be excessive weight gain while the mother is pregnant, older age of the mother, and amniocentesis, a diagnostic procedure in which amniotic fluid is withdrawn from the amniotic sac. This procedure can detect fetal abnormalities. Unfortunately, amniocentesis causes a slightly increased incidence of miscarriage, as well as rupture of the membranes.

As with cardiovascular complications, treating diabetic kidney damage (nephropathy) may include controlling high blood pressure, which can be treated with drugs, according to Maria Thomas and Loren W. Greene, MD.[12]

"You may want to reduce salt intake, reduce your potassium intake and increase your calcium intake," the authors said. "Calcium supplements, as well as vitamin D supplements, may be necessary if kidney disease progresses. As we know, healthy kidneys produce active vitamin D."

Writing in *Clinical Pearls,* Kirk Hamilton published his interview with Barbara J. Boucher, MD, of the Royal London School of Medicine and Dentistry in England, concerning vitamin D and glucose intolerance. Boucher said that vitamin D is needed by the islet cells to secrete insulin normally. This may happen because vitamin D helps ensure an adequate supply of calcium, upon which many enzymes related to insulin secretion and release are dependent.[13]

Boucher and her colleagues reported that vitamin D is directly related to the capacity to secrete insulin and inversely related to glucose tolerance. In a previous study, they said that elderly Dutchmen had a vitamin D deficiency of 39 percent and that glucose tolerance was more advanced in those with the least vitamin D. They also said that vitamin D status related inversely to insulin sensitivity and that, in those depleted of insulin, or in whom it is not being produced in adequate amounts, it increases the risk of becoming diabetic.

Boucher added that, in animal studies, there is considerable evidence that vitamin D supplements can improve insulin secretion in the islets of the pancreas. In addition, vitamin D supplements given to humans over a considerable period can improve insulin secretion and glucose tolerance in those who have osteomalacia, since these patients are severely deficient in vitamin D.

Vitamin D can improve insulin resistance by reducing hyperinsulinemia (high levels of insulin in the blood), along with improving glucose tolerance when given in the early stages of glucose intolerance in kidney disease, Boucher added. The latter develops when vitamin D is not properly formed.

In an article in *Diabetes Care,* a research team at Tufts–New England Medical Center in Boston, and other facilities, said that taking vitamin D and calcium from supplements instead of diet was significantly associated with a lower risk of type 2 diabetes. This was said to be the first prospective study to suggest that the two nutrients may reduce the risk of type 2 diabetes in women, according to Anastassios G. Pittas, MD, the lead researcher.[14]

If these results can be confirmed in further studies, they will have important public health implications, since these two nutrients can be implemented easily and inexpensively to prevent type 2 diabetes, the researchers added.

As an example, women who consumed 800 IU/day or more of vitamin D had a 23 percent lower risk of developing diabetes when compared to women who consumed 200 IU/day. And women who consumed 1,200 mg/day of calcium had a 21 percent lower risk of developing diabetes than those who were getting less than 600 mg/day.

At Aker and Ulleval University Hospitals and the Norwegian Institute of Public Health in Oslo, Lars C. Stene and colleagues reported that, in Norway, cod liver oil is an important source of dietary vitamin D, along with the long-chain omega-3 fatty acids eisosapentaenoic acid and docosahexaenoic acid, all of which have biological properties of potential relevance for the prevention of type 1 diabetes in children.[15]

"Type 1 diabetes is among the most preventable chronic diseases with onset in childhood, which results from an immune mediated destruction of pancreatic B cells and is linked to genes in the human lymphocyte antigens (HLA) complex on chromosome 6p21," the researchers said. "However, genetic susceptibility is not sufficient for development of the disease."

Although the environmental triggers of the disease are unknown, early diet is among the strongest candidates, along with viral infections, they added. Theories have been investigated on the role of breastfeeding and the timing of the introduction of cow's milk into the infant's diet. Other aspects of diet have also been investigated, including nitrosamines, and the consumption of fat, proteins, and meat.

A few studies have focused on the immunomodulatory effects of vitamin D, which may be relevant in the prevention of type 1 diabetes. After the vitamin was found to prevent autoimmune diabetes in nondiabetic mice, two studies revealed an association between the use of vitamin D supplements in the first year of life and a lower risk of type 1 diabetes.

"Cod liver oil is an important source of both vitamin D and omega-3 fatty acids in the Norwegian population," the researchers added. "In Norway, dietary vitamin D supplementation is recommended from infancy, preferably in the form of cod liver oil. Omega-3 fatty acids are incorporated into cell membranes and have anti-inflammatory properties that may be relevant for the prevention of type 1 diabetes, such as decreased expression of HLA class II molecules on activated human monocytes and reduced expression of interleukin 1-Beta."

It is estimated that 5 million Americans and 10 million Europeans have congestive heart failure, reported Stefanie S. Schleithoff and colleagues at the University of Bonn in Germany and other facilities. They said that their study found that vitamin D can serve as an anti-inflammatory agent and may be useful in the management of congestive heart failure. Also, the vitamin was able to suppress blood levels of parathyroid hormone, a hormone that may contribute to impaired cardiac function.[16]

Commenting on the study in the *American Journal of Clinical Nutrition,* Reinhold Vieth and Samantha Kimball of the University of Toronto and Mount Sinai Hospital in Canada, said that congestive heart failure can be caused by diabetes, high blood pressure, coronary artery disease, or defective heart valves.[17]

The just-cited German study is important, Vieth and Kimball said, because it offers two insights about the functions of vitamin D. First, the article confirms that vitamin D supplementation affects immune-modulating cytokines in desirable ways, and second, it suggests that a higher recommended dose of the vitamin is needed. Cytokines are hormones that regulate the intensity and duration of immune suppression.

A study by K. K. Witte and A. L. Clark revealed that 400 IU/day of vitamin D was not effective in cytokine concentrations; however, another study by B. D. Mahon and colleagues, using 1,000 IU/day of the vitamin, produced modest results, the Canadian researchers pointed out. However, in the Schleithoff et al study, the research team used 2,000 IU/day of vitamin D, which produced more substantial results on inflammatory cytokine concentrations. Higher doses of the vitamin also have greater effects on regulatory molecules of the immune system.

Writing in the *American Journal of Clinical Nutrition,* Robert P. Heaney, MD, and colleagues at Creighton University in Omaha, reported that it has long been recognized that vitamin D is not a nutrient in the usual sense, since it is not naturally present in most of the foods our ancestors would have consumed.[18]

Evolving in equatorial East Africa, human beings would have received generous amounts of radiation from the sun and, consequently, high amounts of vitamin D year-round. It has also been recognized that people living in northern latitudes or in environments in which they are deprived of solar exposure need vitamin D supplements, the researchers added. Healthy men seem to use 3,000 to 5,000 IU/day of cholecalciferol (D_3), which meets over 80 percent of their winter cholecalciferol needs.

14.

Gum Disease

The gums are the soft tissue that cover the alveolar bone and are continuous with the mucous membrane of the mouth, lips, and cheeks, reported *The Book of Health*. Their blood supply comes from the vessels of the jaws and face. They respond to injury just as other mucous membranes of the body do.[1]

A weak place in the anatomical arrangement of these tissues is the line of junction of the gum margin around the back of the teeth, the publication said. During eruption, the tooth moves through the gum until it emerges into the mouth. As it comes through, the tooth loses its intact epithelial covering.

"The gingival tissues adapt closely to the necks of the teeth and form a working seal due to the strength of the connective tissue fibers in the edge of the gum," the publication added. "Covering epithelium lines the tooth side of the gingiva for a short distance. As the mucous membranes secrete, tooth and gum are covered by mucoid substances that keep the surface slippery. These shiny secretions aid passage of foods during chewing and swallowing and they help to keep the mouth clean as they flow slowly from the tissues over the teeth and through the mouth into the throat."

Although dental caries are the principal cause of tooth loss before age thirty-five, periodontal disease is responsible for most loose teeth and 70 percent of the tooth loss after the age of forty, according to the *Columbia University College of Physicians and Surgeons Complete Home Medical Guide*.[2]

Periodontal disease occurs in the periodontium, that is, the gums (gingivae), the periodontal ligament, and the alveolar bone that together make up the supporting structure of the teeth.

"There are several types of periodontal disease, but they have one thing in common: They all lead to the destruction of the structures surrounding the teeth. As with caries, bacterial plaque is an underlying cause of periodontal disease, although the kinds of bacteria and the destructive process are different," the publication said.

Gingivitis is a superficial inflammation of the gum tissue, due to irritation by bacterial products in the plaque. The first sign of gingivitis is red, swollen gums, which bleed easily when subjected to pressure. This is especially noticeable with tooth brushing.

As we know, vitamin D plays a significant role in calcium homeostasis, and it is essential for both growth and preservation; however, more recently, anti-inflammatory effects of the vitamin have been described in the literature, according to Thomas Dietrich at the Boston University Goldman School of Dental Medicine in Massachusetts and colleagues at other facilities. As an example, 1,25-dihydroxyvitamin D_3 ($1,25(OH)_2D_3$) was shown to inhibit antigen-induced T-cell proliferation and cytokine production.[3]

In animal studies, beneficial effects of the vitamin and its analogs were found for various autoimmune diseases. In epidemiological studies, inverse associations between intake of vitamin D and incidence of multiple sclerosis and type 1 diabetes have been documented.

"Some studies have suggested that vitamin D may have beneficial effects on periodontal disease and tooth loss, possibly because of its anti-inflammatory effects," Dietrich said. "Another common dental health problem, prevalent across all ages, is chronic marginal gingivitis, a chronic inflammation of the gingival tissues that is induced by bacterial dental plaque. In susceptible people, the gingival inflammation may eventually lead to the destruction of periodontal ligament and alveolar bone and it may then evolve into periodontal disease" (E. A. Krall et al., "Calcium and Vitamin D Supplements Reduce Tooth Loss in the Elderly," *American Journal of Medicine* 111 [2001]: 452–456; and T. Dietrich et al., "Association between Serum Concentrations of 25-Hydroxyvitamin D and Periodontal Disease in the U.S. Population," *American Journal of Clinical Nutrition* 80 [2004]: 108–113, which will be discussed later).

The research team analyzed data from 77,503 gingival units (teeth) in 6,700 never-smokers, ranging in age from thirteen to over ninety, from the Third National Health and Nutrition Examination Survey. The researchers adjusted for age, sex, race/ethnicity, body mass index, diabetes, use of oral contraceptives and hormone replacement therapy among women, intake of vitamin C, missing teeth, full-crown coverage, presence of calculus, frequency of dental visits, and dental examiner and survey data.

The research team found that, compared with sites in those in the lowest 25(OH)D quintile intake of the vitamin, sites in those in the highest 25(OH)D quintile were 20 percent less likely to bleed on gingival probing. The association, which appeared to be linear over the entire 25(OH)D range, was consistent across a racial or ethnic group and was similar among men and women, as well as among users and nonusers of vitamin and mineral supplements.

Because bone loss is pathognomonic for periodontal disease, studies have linked vitamin D status and polymorphisms of the vitamin D receptor genes to periodontal disease and tooth loss, the researchers added. In NHANES III, they reported an inverse association between blood concentrations of 25(OH)D and the prevalence of periodontal disease, as measured by periodontal attachment loss. The results of the present study are consistent with an anti-inflammatory effect of vitamin D on gingival inflammation, which may be alternative pathways by which the vitamin may be beneficial for the prevention of periodontal disease. NHANES III was the National Health and Nutrition Examination Survey, conducted in 1993, which showed what had happened to cholesterol levels among U.S. adults in the twelve years from 1978 to 1990.

"The results of the present study suggest that increased serum concentrations of vitamin D may be beneficial in regard to gingivitis susceptibility," the researchers concluded. "This inverse association may be due to the anti-inflammatory effect of vitamin D, which may be present in blood concentrations of 25(OH)D greater than 90 to 100 nmol/l."

In an article in the *American Journal of Clinical Nutrition,* mentioned earlier, many of the same researchers reported that periodontal disease is a primary cause of tooth loss, especially in the elderly.[4]

"Periodontal disease and associated tooth loss affect the quality of life, dietary quality, and nutrient intake, and recent reports found associations between periodontal disease and increased risks of cardiovascular disease," the researchers added. "Possible mechanisms involved in these associations are depressed dietary quality and chronic inflammation."

The periodontal tissue destruction observed in periodontal disease is widely accepted as being host-mediated through the release of pro-inflammatory cytokines by local tissues and immune cells to respond to bacteria of dental plaque and their products and metabolites, the researchers continued. These cytokines have the potential to stimulate bone resorption in a receptive host, which may be most pronounced among those with low bone density. Actually, several studies have reported positive associations between osteoporosis or low bone density and alveolar bone and tooth loss, indicating that poor overall bone quality may be a risk factor for periodontal disease.

The researchers added that vitamin D might affect periodontal disease both through an effect on bone mineral density and through immunomodulatory effects. The vitamin is well-established as being essential for bone growth and preservation. For example, in the elderly, supplemental vitamin D and calcium are effective in preventing nonvertebral fractures.

A potential anti-inflammatory effect of vitamin D has been indicated by an increasing amount of data suggesting that the active metabolite of 25-hydroxyvitamin D—1,25-dihydroxyvitamin D—has been found to inhibit cytokine production and cell proliferation. One study has suggested that supplemental vitamin D and calcium may significantly reduce tooth loss in the elderly over a three-year period.

In their 2004 study, the researchers analyzed data on periodontal attachment loss (AL) and blood levels of $25(OH)D_3$ in 11,202 people over the age of twenty. The model was stratified by age and sex, and it was adjusted for age within age groups, race or ethnicity, smoking habits, diabetes, poverty/income ratio, body mass index, estrogen use, and gingival bleeding.

The research team reported that $25(OH)D_3$ concentrations were significantly and inversely associated with AL in both men and women over the age of fifty. Compared with men in the highest $25(OH)D_3$ quintile, those in the lowest quintile had a mean AL that was 0.39 millimeter (95 percent) higher. In women, the difference in AL between the lowest and highest quintiles of intake was 0.26 millimeter. In men and women younger than fifty, there was no significant association between $25(OH)D_3$ and AL.

"Low serum $25(OH)D_3$ concentrations may be associated with periodontal disease independently of body mass index," the researchers concluded. "Given the high prevalence of periodontal disease and vitamin D deficiency these findings may have important public health implications."

15.

Immunity

An elaborate, finely tuned defense system destroys and counters the effects of viruses, bacteria, yeasts, and foreign substances that operate within the tissues and cells in the bloodstream. Called the immune system, this system distinguishes *self* from *nonself;* that is, substances that are not part of the body, according to Robert A. Ronzio, PhD.[1]

"When the immune system is healthy, it destroys foreign elements without causing symptoms, but an imbalanced immune system can set the stage for disease," he said. "Foreign substances and microorganisms may not be recognized or destroyed, resulting in chronic infection. An imbalanced immune system can attack the body's own tissues, creating autoimmune diseases, or it can over-respond to common substances, thereby creating allergies."

Cellular immunity includes macrophages, cells that engulf foreign invaders, Ronzio said. Macrophages live in the tissues like the spleen, the liver (Kupffer cells), the lymph nodes (wandering macrophages), the spinal cord, the brain (microglia), and connective tissue.

Lymphocytes are an important type of white blood cell, he continued. T-cells are highly specialized lymphocytes that attack viruses, tumors, and transplanted cells that regulate the immune system. T-cells are produced by the thymus gland and they work with B-cells, which produce defensive proteins called antibodies.

"Certain T–helper cells, acting as 'generals,' read antigens—defensive proteins—and, in turn, stimulate the production of specialized T–killer cells, which are foot soldiers that destroy abnormal cells or foreign materials," Ronzio added.

The different types of immune cells communicate with each other via lymphokines or protein messengers. As an example, macrophages produce a lymphokine called interleukin-1 to activate T–helper cells and they, in turn, produce interleukin-2, which stimulate the production of the killer T-cells. Helper T-cells also produce gamma interferon, which activates killer T-cells.

Mast cells are a type of T-cell that thrives in tissues and fights local infection, Ronzio said. These cells also release special chemicals like histamine, as well as various lymphokines that trigger inflammation marked by swelling (edema); reduce redness; and cause itching, sneezing, and runny nose. Lymphokines also trigger phagocytes (macrophages), which destroy foreign matter and dispose of signal proteins once they have served their purpose.

Antibodies (gamma globulins) are Y-shaped proteins designed to target a particular antigen. An antibody can neutralize the foreign substance either by binding to it or by targeting it for attack by other cells and chemicals.

"B cells, which originate in bone marrow, are a type of lymphocyte that yield plasma cells, which are specialized to produce antibodies when exposed to foreign invaders," Ronzio said. "B cell proliferation, maturation, and antibody production are stimulated by T-helper infected cells. Another type of cell, T suppressor cells, gear down the immune system by turning off B cell production. Thus, T suppressor cells limit allergic attacks and autoimmune reactions."

A research team from Finland, reporting in the *American Journal of Clinical Nutrition* in 2007, investigated the role of vitamin D on the immunity involved in combating acute respiratory infections. The study involved eight hundred young men engaged in military service who were based in southern Finland in July 2002.[2]

"On the basis of the present study's finding that low vitamin D status at initial entry into military service and subsequent respiratory infections are statistically significantly related, it seems evident that vitamin D insufficiency contributes to proneness to these diseases," said Ilkka Laaksi of the University of Tampere in Finland, the lead researcher, and colleagues throughout Finland. Taking into account the geographical position of Finland, which extends from the 60th to the 70th northern parallel, the researchers expected to see regional differences in the soldiers' vitamin D concentrations. However, they found no significant difference in serum 25(OH)D concentrations between subjects from northern and southern Finland.

However, in the study, in which the men were followed for six months and the days missed from duty because of respiratory infections were analyzed, it was found that those with blood levels of 25(OH)D of less than 40 nmol/l had significantly more days absent from duty due to respiratory infections than did the controls. They also found a lower amount of vitamin D in the blood of men who smoked.

"The findings from our study contribute to the diversity of consequences already known to result from vitamin D insufficiency and recognized as carrying significant global public health implications," Laaksi said. "In the context of immune function, clarification of the role of vitamin D in relation to infections, such as acute respiratory infections, represents a high priority for future research."

In an article in *The Experts Speak,* Kirk Hamilton interviewed F. Michael Gloth III, MD, of Union Memorial Hospital in Baltimore, concerning vitamin D, immunity, and the elderly. Gloth said that a study published in the *Lancet* found that 36 percent of elderly men and 47 percent of elderly women had low levels of vitamin D in their blood.[3]

Gloth added that a vitamin D deficiency has been associated with bone loss and increased risk of fractures, muscle weakness, pain, and impairment of immunological function. In addition, there is a link between vitamin D and diminished function of white blood cells, as well as a link between the vitamin and cellular differentiation; that is, posession of one or more functions different from the original diagnosis.

While a debate continues on the proper dosage of vitamin D for the elderly, Gloth and his colleagues recommend either 100,000 IU every three months or 800–1,000 IU/day, for those who are sunlight-deprived.

"This is a maintenance schedule," Gloth continued, "and if someone is vitamin D deficient, it would be worthwhile giving larger doses, such as 50,000 to 100,000 IU two or three times during the first week and then placing the patient on maintenance dosing."

The researchers recommend either vitamin D_2 (ergocalciferol) or vitamin D_3 (cholecalciferol). This form goes through some conversion until it reaches the kidneys, where it is converted to the most active form, the 1,25-dihydroxyvitamin D metabolite.

"It is of interest to report that some people who have severe kidney disease are not able to manufacture enough of the most active metabolite (1,25-dihydroxyvitamin D), so the recommendation is to give that form of the vitamin," Gloth continued. "When this is done, particular attention needs to be addressed to monitoring calcium levels. Adverse events are probably more likely with this form of supplementation and, for this reason, the type of supplementation is reserved for those who have severe kidney disease. Vitamin D_2 and vitamin D_3 are thought to be equal in bioavailability in humans. But if you have rickets, that is a different story."

Gloth went on to say that, although changes occur with age and the skin's ability to manufacture the active forms of vitamin D, it is reasonable to expect that thirty minutes of sunlight two or three times a week should lead to adequate vitamin D levels. However, it is noteworthy to mention that the wavelength necessary to convert precursor molecules to vitamin D is blocked by glass, so sitting in a solarium provides no benefit with regard to vitamin D.

In an article in *Pediatric Infectious Disease Journal,* researchers reviewed the potential immune-stimulating effects of vitamin D and other nutrients. The studies suggest that Th_1-Th_2 may be an important regulatory mechanism by which micronutrients have an impact on immune response. For example, the presence or absence of specific micronutrients during the development of the T–helper cell subpopulation influence whether a Th_1 or Th_2 type response becomes deficient. *Th* is an abbreviation for T–helper cells.[4]

The research team added that the strongest evidence suggests that vitamin A and vitamin D_3 suppress a Th_1 response and promote a Th_2 response. Prostaglandin E_2 is a potent stimulator of the Th_2 response and suppresses the Th_1 response.

In addition, vitamins C and E increase dehydroepiandrosterone production, and retinol (vitamin A) may increase the production of cortisol, which may affect immune function. Vitamin D_3 (calcitriol) may play a similar role to that of cortisol, the researchers added.

The use of vitamins to modify the Th_1-Th_2 response might be an important tool in reducing childhood morbidity in developing countries, the researchers continued.

An altered nutritional status can have a profound effect on the immune system and on behavior, explained John E. Morley, MB, of St. Louis University School of Medicine in Missouri. For example, protein-energy undernutrition and aging result in similar changes in immune function. Calorie supplementation has been shown to enhance delayed skin hypersensitivity in older, poorly nourished individuals.[5]

He added that calorie supplementation has normalized CD_4 and CD_8 cells close to values in healthy individuals. A vitamin D deficiency, which can occur even in the elderly living in sunny climates, has been shown to play a role in macrophage function and, in particular, to be important in allowing the appro-

priate killing of *Mycobacterium tuberculosis. CD* refers to "cluster of c
tiation." Cell membrane molecules are used to classify leukocytes into subsets,
and CD molecules are classified by monoclonal antibodies. Thus, CD_4 is an
abbreviation for "cluster of differentiation 4." CD_8 refers to an abbreviation for
"cluster of differentiation 8."

Morley said that a one-year trial of vitamin-mineral supplementation in the
elderly decreased infection rate and enhanced natural killer cell activity, mitogen-
induced T-cell proliferation activity, and interleukin-2 production.

Writing in *Clinical Pearls,* Kirk Hamilton interviewed Margherita T. Cantorna, PhD, of University Park, Pennsylvania, who suggested that vitamin D may
be related to autoimmune diseases. For example, vitamin D levels are low in
those with autoimmune diseases. A deficiency in the vitamin exacerbates symptoms of autoimmune disease, such as multiple sclerosis, at least in experimental animals. And, she added, the hormonally active form of the vitamin
ameliorates symptoms of these diseases.[6]

She goes on to say that vitamin D has been shown to decrease the number
and function of T-cells, which cause autoimmune diseases. In experiments
involving animal models, symptoms improved in lupus, multiple sclerosis, type
1 diabetes, and arthritis when vitamin D therapy was administered.

There are clearly secondary benefits of vitamin D supplementation, she said.
As an example, many patients with autoimmune diseases have low bone mass,
which increases the risk of bone fractures.

"If the vitamin D hypothesis is true, then any population which is at higher
risk for vitamin D inadequacy would also increase their risk for autoimmune
diseases," she added. "I would suggest increasing consumption of vitamin D
fortified milk to increase vitamin D intake. The milk has other features which
also support bone health."

16.

Multiple Sclerosis

At La Salpetrière in Paris, Jean Martin Charcot (1825–1893), who created one of the greatest modern neurological clinics, identified many previously unknown nervous disorders. He also increased our knowledge of diseases of muscles and the nervous system, many of which bear his name, reported *The Book of Health*.[1]

Charcot was the first to cite the importance of psychological forces in mental disorders. In addition to his brilliant neurological work at the hospital, he is remembered for his scientific study of hypnosis and the many gifted pupils he inspired, including Sigmund Freud.

Charcot initially gave a good medical account of multiple sclerosis (MS) in 1857, when he showed that MS patients had plaques, or patches of hardening, scattered throughout their brains and spinal cords, added Geoffrey Dean, MD, in *Medical and Health Annual*. Charcot referred to the disorder as *sclerose en plaques*. The plaques are caused by the loss of myelin, the fatty material that makes up the sheath covering nerve fibers.[2]

MS is the most common disabling neurological disorder of young adults in the Western world, Dean said. But it seldom occurs before the age of fifteen or sixteen and it reaches its peak in those in their early thirties. The disorder is more common in women than in men, affecting about three women for every two men, and it is typically a disease of exacerbations and remissions.

Among the first symptoms of MS are patches of demyelination in the optic nerves, resulting in blurring of vision in one or both eyes (optic neuritis), Dean continued. This disturbance can last from a few days up to a month or six weeks, after which vision often returns to normal.

"Thirty-five percent of the men and seventy-five percent of the women who have an attack of optic neuritis will go on to develop MS within the next fifteen years," Dean said.

Since MS plaques can occur anywhere in the central nervous system, they can cause sensory symptoms, such as altered sensation in part of the body, loss of muscle power, or ataxia (incoordination of movement). If ataxia is severe, it may cause scanning speech (slow enunciation with a tendency to hesitate at the beginning of a word or syllable).

"Those with MS often fatigue easily," Dean continued. "And some of the patients have a problem with controlling urination. Although sexual function is usually normal, sexual activity may be reduced because of fatigue. Mental functions are generally normal, although depression may occur. However, it should be emphasized that even after MS has been diagnosed, the majority of the patients are well and able to live a normal or near-normal life."

Life expectancy with MS is over thirty years after the disease has been diagnosed. Those with MS do not die from the disease, but the complications, such as immobility, may lead to events or situations that shorten life.

"In the early stages, the diagnosis is often in doubt and the suspicious illness can only be called 'possible MS,' " Dean said. "Typically, there is a delay of several years after the first symptoms appear before a firm diagnosis can be made."

It has now been established that MS results from some combination of genetic and environmental factors, Dean continued. The environmental factors may well be a reaction to one or a number of viral infections, which are most likely to occur during early childhood. Viruses can remain latent in the nervous system throughout life and cause problems only when, for one reason or another, immunity to the virus is lowered.

"A new area of investigation has been opened by the findings of Howard Weiner and David Hafler of the Harvard Medical School in Boston, Massachusetts, who showed, in a double blind study, that MS patients who took capsules containing bovine myelin had fewer attacks of MS than a control group (six out of fifteen in the treatment group had attacks, compared with twelve of fifteen in the control group). This is suggestive evidence that the immune system may be induced to tolerate proteins it considers to be foreign," Dean said.

Multiple sclerosis is among the most common neurological diseases in young adults, affecting 350,000 people in the United States and 2 million worldwide, explained Kassandra L. Munger, MSc, of the Harvard School of Public Health in Boston and colleagues at various facilities.[3]

It is theorized that MS is an autoimmune disease in which an unknown agent or agents triggers a T-cell-mediated inflammatory attack, thereby causing demyelination of central nervous tissue.

"A striking feature of the global distribution of MS is a multifold increase in incidence with increasing latitude, both north and south of the equator," Munger said. "Genetic disposition contributes to the variation, but the change in MS risk with migration among those of common ancestry strongly supports a role for environmental factors. One potential factor may be vitamin D, a potent immunomodulator that in its hormonal form can prevent experimental autoimmune encephalomyelitis (EAE), an animal model of MS."

Since food provides little vitamin D, the major source for most people is through skin exposure to sunlight, she continued. At latitudes of 42 degrees or more (Boston, for example), in winter, most UV-B radiation is absorbed by the atmosphere, and even prolonged sun exposure is insufficient to generate vitamin D.

"A protective effect of vitamin D on MS is supported by the reduced MS risk associated with sun exposure, as well as use of vitamin D supplements, but evidence remains inconclusive," she said. "In the present study, we examined, prospectively, for the first time, whether high blood levels of 25-hydroxyvitamin D, a good marker of vitamin D availability to tissues, predict a lower risk of MS."

The research team used data from more than 7 million U.S. military personnel who had blood samples stored in the Department of Defense Serum Repository. MS cases were identified through Army and Navy physical disability databases for 1992 through 2004, and diagnoses were confirmed by medical record review. Vitamin D status was estimated by averaging 25-hydroxyvitamin D levels of two or more blood samples collected before the date of initial MS symptoms.

The researchers reported that among whites (148 cases and 296 controls), the risk of MS significantly decreased with increasing levels of 25-hydroxyvitamin D. Among blacks and Hispanics (109 cases and 218 controls), who had lower 25-hydroxyvitamin D levels than whites, no significant associations between vitamin D and MS risk were found.

However, the researchers concluded that the results of their study suggests that high circulating levels of vitamin D are associated with a lower risk of MS.

In a study at the University of Wisconsin at Madison, a research team, headed by Colleen E. Hayes, revealed that exogenous (outside the body) 1,25-dihydroxyvitamin D, the hormonal form of vitamin D_3, can completely prevent experimental autoimmune encephalomyelitis, as previously mentioned. The authors are convinced that the chief environmental factor in the causation of MS is the degree of sunlight exposure catalyzing the production of vitamin D_3 in the skin. In their view, the hormonal form of D_3 is a selective immune system regulator that inhibits the autoimmune disease.[4]

The research team added that, under low sunlight conditions, insufficient vitamin D_3 is produced, limiting the production of 1,25-dihydroxyvitamin D_3, which puts people at risk for MS.

While the evidence for vitamin D_3 having a protective environmental effect against MS is circumstantial, it is still compelling, the researchers said. This theory explains the striking geographical distribution of MS, which is almost rare in equatorial regions and whose prevalence increases dramatically with latitude in both hemispheres. This also explains the disparity in MS rates within particular countries. For instance, in Switzerland there is a high incidence of MS at low altitudes and low rates at high altitudes (where UV-light intensity is higher, resulting in greater vitamin D_3 synthesis). By the same token, in Norway, there is a lower prevalence of MS along the coast, where fish are consumed in large amounts (fish oils are rich in vitamin D_3), and a higher incidence inland.

Hayes goes on to say that the various studies open the possibility that MS may be preventable in genetically susceptible people, with early intervention that provides adequate levels of active 1,25-dihydroxyvitamin D or its analogs.

There is much interest in the role of vitamin D_3 in many aspects of health and disease, and the rationale for vitamin D_3 treatment in MS is that metabolites of vitamin D_3 function as paracrine (hormone function) immune modulators, screening the proliferation of pro-inflammatory T-lymphocytes and decreasing the production of cytokines, both of which contribute to the pathogenesis of MS, reported Samantha M. Kimball and colleagues at Mount Sinai Hospital in Toronto.[5]

In patients with congestive heart failure, vitamin D_3 treatment at 2,000 IU/day affected cytokine profiles in a way that would be desirable for those with MS, the researchers said. The seasonal fluctuation in the number of gadolinium-enhancing lesions determined by magnetic resonance imaging tend to be fewest at the time when blood 25(OH)D concentrations are highest. Taken together, the data suggest that vitamin D_3 may play a role in the regulation of clinical disease activity, the researchers added. Cytokines are hormonelike proteins that regulate immune responses. Gadolinium, named after Johan Gadolin, a Finnish chemist, is used in magnetic resonance imaging.

During a twenty-eight-week trial involving twelve patients in an active phase of MS, the patients were given 1,200 mg/day of elemental calcium with progressively increasing doses of vitamin D_3, ranging from 28,000 to 280,000 IU/week.

The research team reported that patients' blood 25(OH)D concentrations reached twice the top of the physiologic range without eliciting hypercalciuria (high amounts of calcium in the blood) or hypercalcuria (excretion of large amounts of calcium in the urine). Thus, their data supports the feasibility of pharmacologic doses of vitamin D_3 for clinical research, and they provide objective evidence that vitamin D intake beyond the current upper limit is safe by a large margin.

At the Helen Hayes Hospital in West Haverstraw, New York, Jeri Nieves, PhD, and colleagues, evaluated eighty women with MS who were admitted to the hospital as part of a research study examining the relationship between vitamin D status and reduced bone mineral density.[6]

Bone mineral density of the lumbar spine and femoral neck was one to two times the standard deviations lower in women with MS, compared with the health reference population. Bone mineral density was lower in those with more severe MS.

It was reported that mean 25-hydroxyvitamin D levels of the sample were 43 nmol/l, which was in the insufficient range, and twenty-three patients had frank vitamin D deficiency of less than 23 nmol/l. Bone mineral density and age-related bone mineral density at skeletal sites measured were lowest where 25-hydroxyvitamin D levels were deficient.

Parathyroid hormone was elevated in thirteen of the patients. Parathyroid hormone levels were more negatively associated with 25-hydroxyvitamin D levels than with bone mineral density.

In addition, dietary intake of vitamin D was below the recommended level in 80 percent of the patients, and 40 percent reported no weekly sunlight exposure. The authors concluded that bone mineral density was significantly reduced in women with MS, which may increase the fracture risk two- or threefold.

Vitamin D deficiency was secondary to hyperparathyroidism and it is probably a significant cause of low mineral density in MS patients, the researchers said. They added that the vitamin D deficiency in female MS patients might be safely and inexpensively corrected with vitamin D supplements. Hyperparathyroidism is a condition that causes elevated blood levels of calcium, decreased blood levels of phosphorus, and an increased excretion of both minerals.

MS has a worldwide prevalence that increases with latitude from the equator both north and south, said G. Dick in the *Journal of the Royal Society of Medicine.* The latitude of a person's place of residence—and the availability of vitamin D—appear to be more of a risk factor than race.[7]

There is a marked tendency for the onset and relapse of MS, such as optic neuritis, peaking in the winter months, he added. There does appear to be an association between MS and upper respiratory tract infection, including sinusitis. Upper respiratory tract infections tend to occur in the winter months and they occur more frequently in colder, wetter, windier latitudes farthest from the equator.

MS is more prevalent in temperate climates than in countries close to the equator, agreed R. A. Hughes of Guy's Hospital in London. Migration before puberty from a high-risk area to a low-risk area can reduce the risk of subsequently developing MS. This suggests that an environmental agent may be a trigger before the individual reaches puberty.[8]

In an article in the *Journal of Women's Health & Gender-Based Medicine,* researchers discussed the various health conditions associated with MS. In 220 women with the disease, between the ages of twenty-three and eighty-one, 47 percent were ambulatory, 38 percent required an assistive walking device, and 15 percent were nonambulatory. Also, 63 percent were premenopausal and 37 percent were postmenopausal.[9]

Risk factors for premature osteoporosis in the premenopausal sample included impaired mobility in 53 percent, corticosteroid use in 82 percent, and vitamin D deficiency as a result of avoidance of sunlight. In addition, 85 percent had never had bone density testing, 50 percent were not taking calcium supplements, and 71 percent were not taking vitamin D.

In the postmenopausal sample, 81 percent had never had bone density testing, 50 percent were not taking calcium supplements, and 70 percent had not received hormone replacement therapy. Only 1 percent were taking bone resorption inhibitors.

Writing in *Neuroepidemiology,* Gary G. Schwartz, PhD, MPH, of the University of Pittsburgh School of Medicine in Pennsylvania, suggests that mortality from MS shows a well-known north–south gradient similar to prostate cancer, both internationally and in the United States. Prostate cancer is now included among the list of diseases whose geographic distribution are significantly correlated with MS. These include colon cancer, dental caries, and Parkinson's disease.[10]

Schwartz goes on to say that these diseases may share an aberration in vitamin D. Evidence demonstrating a multifaceted role of vitamin D in immunoregulation suggests that a vitamin D aberration may contribute to the etiology of MS. The pathogenesis of MS is related to T-cell-mediated events.

Advances in the immunology of vitamin D suggest the following hypothesis for the etiology of MS: MS results from an inflammatory response triggered by exogenous factors, such as viral infections, trauma, or lesions to the central nervous system in genetically susceptible people, he added.

In addition, low levels of biologically active vitamin D may fail to inhibit the inflammatory T-cell response. These activated T-cells interact with neural tissue, thereby resulting in sensitization against neural antigens, or what is called autoimmunization.

In an article in *Archives of Neurology,* Schwartz suggests that calcitriol (vitamin D_3) may help to mediate the protective effect of pregnancy on MS. Pregnancy is associated with a reduction in MS activity, with exacerbations occurring at an increased rate postpartum.[11]

He added that this protective effect of pregnancy may be due to an immunosuppressive factor that increases during pregnancy, but declines after delivery.

Calcitriol may be this immunosuppressive protective factor, he continued. Levels of calcitriol increase gradually during the first trimester of pregnancy, peak during the third trimester, and fall rapidly after delivery.

Vitamin D_3 is an immunomodulator hormone, and its modes of action are similar to immunosuppressant drugs such as cyclosporine. These drugs selectively inhibit T–helper lymphocyte activation, cytokine production, and lymphocyte proliferation, he said. In cultures of peripheral mononuclear cells, calcitriol inhibits nitrogen- and antigen-induced lymphocyte proliferation, and suppresses the production of interleukins-1 and -2, as well as interferon gamma.

Schwartz added that MS is common at latitudes where there is little sunlight, which suggests that the disturbed immunoregulation, due to a deficiency of the vitamin, may play a role in the pathogenesis of MS. Supplementation of vitamin D_3 in women with MS during postpartum periods should inhibit the rebound of clinical disease activity, he said.

17.

Osteoarthritis

A joint disease that is aggravated by mechanical stress, osteoarthritis is characterized by the degeneration of cartilage that lines joints or by osteophyte formation (that is, the formation of bony outgrowths), which results in pain, stiffness, and sometimes loss of function of the affected joint, reported the *American Medical Association Home Medical Encyclopedia*.[1]

"Osteoarthritis occurs in almost all people over the age of 60 and [most], but not all of them, exhibit symptoms," the publication said. "Various factors lead to the development of osteoarthritis earlier in life, including an injury to a joint or a congenital joint deformity. Osteoarthritis may occur with rheumatoid arthritis. Severe osteoarthritis affects 3 times more women than men." (Rheumatoid arthritis is a systemic disease involving chronic and progressive inflammatory involvement of joints as well as atrophy of muscles.)

Patients with osteoarthritis complain of pain, swelling, creaking, and stiffness of one or more joints. These conditions can interfere with walking and dressing, and they can disrupt sleep.

Weakness and shrinkage (atrophy) of surrounding muscles may develop if pain prevents the joint from being used regularly, the publication added. The affected joints become enlarged and distorted by osteophytes, which account for the gnarled appearance of hands affected by the disease.

Osteoarthritis results from excessive wear on joints, and it is sometimes due to obesity or to a slight deformity or misalignment of bones in a joint. The healthy joint is lined with smooth cartilage and lubricated by synovial fluid, but, in osteoarthritis, the cartilage becomes rough and flaky, and pieces drop off to form loose bodies.

The typical sign of degenerative arthritis is the appearance of knobs at the end joints of the first and second fingers, according to *The Book of Health*. These are called Heberden's nodes, and they are an outgrowth (hypertrophy) of bone at the margins of the joint. They differ from those of gout by being immobile because they are attached to the bone, whereas those of gout are freely movable and contain urate crystals. The nodes differ from those of rheumatoid arthritis because in this condition the middle joint is attacked, the swelling is spindle-shaped, and, usually, the joint is hot and shiny.[2]

"Heberden's nodes on the fingers are nine times as common in women as in men," the publication added. "They worry patients because of their unsightliness, rather than because of any functional difficulty, which is rare. The nodes can appear in men following trauma." (The nodes are named after William Heberden [1710–1801], an English physician.)

In evaluating 556 volunteers from the Framingham Study, osteoarthritis was found in seventy-five knees and progressive osteoarthritis in sixty-two knees, as reported in the *Annals of Internal Medicine.* The data revealed that the risk for progression increased threefold in those who were in the middle and lower tertiles for both intake and blood levels of vitamin D, when compared to those who were in the upper levels of intake.[3]

Low blood levels of the vitamin predicted loss of cartilage and osteophyte growth. Low intake and low blood levels of the vitamin appear to be a risk factor for the progression of osteoarthritis of the knee, the publication added.

The Framingham Study, which began in 1949, studied five thousand people in the Massachusetts town, measuring physical activity, cigarette use, body weight, blood pressure, cholesterol levels, and other parameters. For decades they have been followed and studied, and the data correlated with clinical events. Children of the original participants have also been evaluated.[4]

T. E. McAlindon, who was involved in the previously cited *Annals of Internal Medicine* study, said that oxidative stress plays a significant role in osteoarthritis, and antioxidant nutrients may be of benefit, as he reported in *Primary and Secondary Preventive Nutrition.*[5]

Vitamin D may have beneficial effects on cartilage, and the data on vitamin D, chondroitin sulfate, and glucosamine are especially significant, he added. Vitamin D should be taken at 400 IU/day or blood levels should be greater than about 30 ng/ml. Large doses, between 400 and 800 IU/day, appear to be safe, he said.

As reported in *Arthritis and Rheumatism,* hip radiographs of 237 volunteers that were taken an average of eight years apart, showed blood levels of vitamin

D that might be associated with incident changes of radiographic hip osteoarthritis, which can be seen radiographically by cartilage loss.[6]

If low vitamin D levels increase the activity of metalloproteinase enzymes that destroy articular (joint) cartilage, then randomized trials of vitamin D supplementation to prevent the progression of hip and bone osteoarthritis may be necessary, the researchers said.

Overweight people are at an increased risk for osteoarthritis and antioxidants (vitamins C, E, and folic acid—the B vitamin) may protect bone by enhancing the bioavailability of cartilage collagen and proteoglycan molecules, reported McAlindon (previously mentioned).[7]

Suboptimal vitamin D levels may have an adverse effect on calcium metabolism, osteoblast activity, matrix ossification, and bone density, McAlindon reported in *Women's Health in Primary Care.* Low tissue levels of vitamin D may impair the ability of bone to respond optimally to pathophysiological processes in osteoarthritis and predispose the patient to disease progression.

In addition, he said, vitamin D may have a direct effect on chondrocytes in osteoarthritis cartilage, since the vitamin regulates the transition from growth-plate cartilage to bone.

In one study, the risk of progression of osteoarthritis was about threefold for those in the middle and lower tertiles of vitamin D intake and blood levels. A low blood level of the vitamin was also predictive of cartilage loss. Low blood levels of the vitamin, as well as low vitamin D in the diet, were related to a progression of osteoarthritis in the knee.

In another trial involving 237 women, there was an increased risk of joint-space narrowing among those in the lower tertile of serum 25-hydroxyvitamin D, as well as an association with continuous measures of progression. In addition, there was evidence of an increased risk of joint-space narrowing in those in the middle tertile of 25-hydroxyvitamin D.

The second study, as well as findings from the well-known Framingham Study, suggests that vitamin D may be protective with respect to osteoarthritis incidence, at least in the hip, McAlindon continued. Those with the lowest risk were in the highest tertile of 25-hydroxyvitamin D levels over 30 ng/ml.

In studying 143 women with rheumatoid arthritis, it was found that blood levels of calcium were normal, but blood levels of vitamin D were significantly below normal in most of the patients, according to the *Nutrition Report.*[8]

It was found that the serum 25-hydroxyvitamin D concentration was less than 12.5 nmol/l in 16 percent of the women. In the winter months, 73 percent of the women had low blood levels of 1,25-dihydroxyvitamin D. Those with the most aggressive disease were associated with the lowest vitamin D concentrations.

18.

Osteomalacia

Aform of osteoporosis that is associated with severe vitamin D deficiency in the elderly, osteomalacia is the impaired mineralization of newly formed bone matrix, according to an article published by researchers T. S. Dharmarajan and colleagues in *Family Practice Recertification*. In the Framingham Study, it was found in about 6 percent of men and 15 percent of women, ranging in age from sixty-seven to ninety-five, which showed that the volunteers had low 25-hydroxyvitamin D levels. The Framingham Study examined the effects of smoking, obesity, blood pressure, and the like, on the five thousand residents of the Massachusetts town from 1949 to 1969.[1]

It was suggested that over half of the community-dwelling, homebound elderly have low blood levels of vitamin D, and this problem is especially critical for institutionalized elderly.

The researchers said that, in one study, up to 40 percent of patients with hip fractures had low levels of vitamin D in their blood. Osteomalacia is characterized as excess osteoid tissue accumulating in undermineralized bone matrix, which reduces the mineral-to-matrix ratio, which should be about 2:1. *Osteoid* means relating to or resembling bone. It is newly formed bone matrix prior to calcification.

It has been well established that impaired bone mineralization weakens bone and can cause deformities and fractures. In osteoporosis, the mineral-to-matrix ratio is generally preserved. However, levels of vitamin D, calcium, and phosphorus, as well as alkaline phosphatase, are typically abnormal in osteomalacia, while being normal in osteoporosis.

In vitamin D deficiency, they added, there is an impairment of calcium absorption, which triggers a rise in parathyroid hormone levels. This increase precedes the development of osteomalacia, which is characterized by normal matrix synthesis by osteoblasts coupled with impaired mineralization. Osteoblasts are bone-forming cells.

The authors go on to say that the excess mineralized bone and increased bone turnover create an irregular trabecular structure that causes deformities and fractures. In advanced cases, osteoblasts may become flattened and halt the forming of new matrix. This results in an overall loss of bone volume. Trabecula are bundles of supporting fibers.

Osteomalacia is known for its deficiencies in vitamin D, calcium, and phosphorus, and the recommended dietary intakes for vitamin D are 400 IU/day for those over fifty and 600 IU/day for anyone over seventy. The ability to absorb calcium decreases with age, especially for those older than seventy, the researchers continued.

While 60–90 percent of dietary vitamin D is absorbed in the upper small intestine, this also declines with age. In addition, the thinning of the skin can reduce the level of the vitamin D precursor, 7-dehydrocholesterol.

Osteomalacia may also be connected with the various drugs that are prescribed for tranquilizing, hypnotic, and antiseizure uses, and anticonvulsants, which are designed to prevent seizures. Some of the older bisphosphonates, especially etidronate disodium, especially in higher dosages, were found to inhibit bone mineralization and cause osteomalacia, the researchers continued. However, this has not been reported in the newer bisphosphonates.

It is estimated that 20 percent of those with osteomalacia cannot walk or can only do so with a limp, and almost half have a waddling gait. Some levels of 25-hydroxyvitamin D are the gold standard for evaluating vitamin D status, and blood levels of 1,25-dihydroxyvitamin D can be misleading, the researchers said. Thus, the goal for treating osteomalacia is to remineralize bone without producing hypervitaminosis D and toxic levels of calcium.

The researchers added that hypervitamininosis D (a deficiency in the vitamin) can be treated with supplemental vitamin D at 800–4,000 IU/day for one to two weeks, followed by a maintenance dose of 400–800 IU/day. Doses of 50,000 IU once a month and, in some cases, 100,000 IU every six months, may be given to ensure adequate levels of vitamin D in the elderly.

Osteomalacia is caused by an insufficient amount of vitamin D in the diet (lack of milk, butter, eggs, or fish liver oils), insufficient exposure to sunlight, or inadequate absorption of the vitamin from the intestine, according to the *American Medical Association Home Medical Guide.* This may be caused by celiac sprue or by intestinal surgery. Rare cases are accompanied by kidney failure, acidosis (increased acidity of body fluids), and certain metabolic disorders that are inherited. Dark-skinned immigrants living in a country that has much less sunlight than their native countries are also at risk.[2]

"Osteomalacia causes pain in the bones, especially in the neck, legs, hips, and ribs; muscle weakness and, if the blood level of calcium is low, tetany (muscle spasms) in the hands, feet, and throat," the publication added.

The suggestion that 200 IU/day of vitamin D may prevent osteomalacia in the absence of sunlight has been proposed, but more of the vitamin is needed to prevent osteoporosis and secondary hyperparathyroidism (an increase in the secretion of the parathyroids, causing an increased secretion of calcium and decreased levels of phosphorus), according to Reinhold Vieth of the University of Toronto and Mount Sinai Hospital in Canada. Other benefits of vitamin D supplementation include preventing some forms of cancer and slowing the progression of osteoarthritis, multiple sclerosis, and high blood pressure.[3]

"If vitamin D is similar to a drug, then dose-finding studies are needed to use it properly, especially if non-classical benefits are potentially relevant," Vieth said. "Alternatively, if by analogy with other nutrients, adult daily reference intake of 200 IU/day is woefully inadequate."

In evaluating two cases of vitamin D–deficient osteomalacia with secondary hyperparathyroidism, A. V. G. Taylor and P. H. Wise reported that, in both instances, vitamin D therapy elevated calcium levels but failed to normalize parathyroid hormone levels, suggesting autonomous (self-contained) parathyroid activity, as they reported the *British Medical Journal*.[4]

Prolonged osteomalacia is associated with autonomous hyperparathyroidism, which may only become apparent with vitamin D replacement therapy. The research team added that it is necessary to monitor blood levels of calcium during treatment for osteomalacia.

19.

Osteoporosis

Osteoporosis, or porous bone, is a major public health threat for an estimated 44 million Americans, or 55 percent of those fifty years of age and older, according to the National Osteoporosis Foundation in Washington, D.C. Currently, 10 million people are estimated to have the disease already, and almost 34 million more are said to have low bone mass, thereby placing them at risk for osteoporosis.[1]

Of the 10 million Americans estimated to have osteoporosis, 8 million are women and 2 million are men. The estimated national direct care expenditures—hospitals, nursing homes, and outpatient services—for osteoporosis fractures was $18 billion in 2002, and costs are continuing to rise.

The foundation added that osteoporosis is responsible for over 1.5 million fractures annually, including:

- Over 300,000 hip fractures

- 700,000 vertebral fractures

- 250,000 wrist fractures

- 300,000 fractures at other sites

Women with a hip fracture are at a fourfold greater risk of incurring a second one, and the risk factors are similar to those for the first hip fracture. Hip fracture risk is increasing most rapidly among Hispanic women, the foundation said.

"By about age twenty, the average woman has acquired 98 percent of her skeletal mass," the foundation said. "Building strong bones during childhood and adolescence can be the best defense against developing osteoporosis later.

153

Also, women can lose up to 20 percent of their bone mass in the five to seven years following menopause, making them more susceptible to osteoporosis. Specialized tests called bone mineral density (BMD) tests can measure bone density in various sites of the body."

Certain people are more likely to develop osteoporosis than others, the foundation continued. Risk factors for osteoporosis include:

1. Personal history of fracture after age fifty.

2. Current low bone mass.

3. History of fracture in a close relative.

4. Being female.

5. Being thin and/or having a small frame.

6. Advanced age.

7. A family history of osteoporosis.

8. Estrogen deficiency as a result of menopause, especially early-onset or surgically induced.

9. Abnormal absence of menstrual periods (amenorrhea).

10. Anorexia nervosa.

11. Low lifetime calcium intake.

12. Vitamin D deficiency.

13. Use of certain medications: corticosteroids, chemotherapy, anticonvulsants, and others.

14. Presence of certain chronic medical conditions.

15. Low testosterone levels in men.

16. An inactive lifestyle.

17. Current cigarette smoking.

18. Excessive use of alcohol.

19. Being Caucasian or Asian, although African Americans and Hispanic Americans are at a significant risk as well.

Osteoporosis is mainly a disease of aging, which involves a decrease in bone tissue mass, according to the *Physicians' Manual for Patients*. Bone is not an inert tissue, but rather one that is constantly rebuilt and reabsorbed in a complex way. Thus, bone requires calcium, vitamin D, phosphorus, hormones, and a proper environment.[2]

"A hormone, estrogen, promotes and participates in the uptake of calcium into bone, while other hormones and chemicals—parathyroids and corticosteroids—promote calcium loss," the publication said. "Calcitonin, a hormone secreted by the thyroid gland, controls bone resorption, that is, the loss of a substance—in this case bone—through physiological or pathological means. Bone loss is thought to be the inevitable consequence of aging; however, in osteoporosis, bone loss considerably exceeds bone formation."

Although the exact causes of osteoporosis are still being debated, there appear to be a number of contributing factors, the publication continued. Hormonal imbalance, which affects the uptake of calcium and phosphorus, seems to be prominent among them. Other causes include an inadequate supply of protein, minerals, and vitamins over a number of years.

Osteoporosis is said to be a "silent" disease, in that it remains undisclosed until a fracture occurs. The initial symptom is often severe lower back pain, aggravated by carrying something heavy. The pain is due to the spontaneous collapse (crush fracture) of one or more of the spinal vertebrae. After a few days, the pain may subside.

"In time," the publication added, "the continued collapse of the vertebrae causes the loss of height and the curvature of the spine that is commonly referred to as 'widow's hump.' In the later stages, there is often chronic, aching pain in the lower back due to the stress of the muscles and ligaments attached to the spine."

A hip fracture that results from a minor fall is another sign that osteoporosis is present. Hip fractures are especially common among elderly white women. Five of every one thousand white women, aged sixty-five to seventy-five, suffer these fractures annually.

"For elderly patients with osteoporosis, precautions should be taken to avoid accidental falls," the publication said. "If glasses are necessary for general vision, they should always be worn. A walking stick or frame should be used if the patient's gait is at all unsteady. Shoes and slippers should have skid resistant soles. And it is wise to install handrails in bathrooms and sturdy banister rails along the stairs."

In the 1930s, when doctors routinely performed autopsies, they noticed that, inside the bones, deep in the marrow, people had grown fat cells, reported Gina

Kolata in the *New York Times*. The older they were, the more their bones were filled with fat.[3]

People did not pay much attention to this discovery, added Clifford J. Rosen, MD, of the Maine Center for Osteoporosis Research and Education and the Jackson Laboratory in Bangor, Maine. They just thought it was part of the aging process.

More recently, scientists have discovered there is a stem cell in bone marrow that can turn into fat or bone, depending on what signals it receives, Kolata continued.

"In osteoporosis," she said, "bone cavities that everyone thought were just empty spaces are actually crammed with fat and patients with osteoporosis have more fat in their bones than people the same age who do not have the bone weakening disease. Other factors that lead to bone loss—steroids, taken to suppress the immune system, bed rest, and removal of a woman's ovaries—also lead to an accumulation of fat in the bones."

As noted by Kolata, this prompted Jane E. Aubin, MD, of the University of Toronto to ask: "Could osteoporosis be prevented or reversed by pushing stem cells to become bone instead of fat?"

While it is intriguing to think that the high levels of fat in bone may be as much a sign of bone weakness and deterioration as low bone density, that notion is still very much a hypothesis, added Jeffrey Gimble, MD, of the Pennington Research Center in Baton Rouge, Louisiana, as cited in Kolata's *New York Times* article. Other explanations include the possibility that fat is needed to strengthen bones.

Gimble added that what makes a strong bone is not necessarily how much calcium it contains, but what's in its center. If a bone was hollow, it would be more brittle, so you have to fill it with something—like fat.

"In the meantime," Kolata added, "scientists are trying to find out what signals drive bone marrow cells along a pathway to become fat or bone. They are also asking whether once cells turn into fat, is it possible to reverse the process and convert them to bone instead?"

In a lengthy article in the February 14, 2001, issue of the *Journal of the American Medical Association,* it was reported that a one-year mortality rate following a hip fracture is about one in five. Unfortunately, as many as two-thirds of hip fracture patients never regain their postoperative capabilities.[4]

Early surgical intervention to address hip fractures brings improved outcomes and decreased perioperative morbidity. Risk factors for low bone mass include being female, being white, increased age, estrogen deficiency, low weight and body mass index, a family history of osteoporosis, smoking, and a history of prior fractures, the researchers added.

In addition, late menarche, early menopause, and low endogenous estrogen production have all been associated with low bone mineral density. In men, 30–60 percent of osteoporosis cases are due to secondary causes, with the most common being hypogonadism (failure of the testes to develop properly), use of glucocorticoids (steroids), and alcoholism.

The researchers added that exercise, especially in later life, even beyond ninety years of age, can increase muscle mass and strength more than twofold. Exercise has also been shown to reduce the risk of falls by about 25 percent. Calcium and vitamin D intake regulate age-related increases in parathyroid hormone levels and bone resorption, although low levels of 25-hydroxyvitamin D are common in seniors and are significantly reduced in cases of hip and other vertebral fractures.

Speaking at the 21st Annual Public Health Nutrition Update Conference, April 12–13, 1995, at the William and Ida Friday Continuing Education Center in Chapel Hill, North Carolina, Michael F. Holick, PhD, MD, of the Boston University School of Medicine, said there is a "silent epidemic" of vitamin D deficiency in the elderly in the United States and this is of serious concern because it increases the risk for skeletal fractures. He added that it is estimated that 30–40 percent of elderly patients with hip fractures are vitamin D–deficient or vitamin D–insufficient.[5]

While the 1995 RDA for vitamin D for adults was 5 mcg (200 IU/day), Holick said there is increasing evidence that this level of the vitamin is insufficient to meet the needs of people who are not exposed to sunlight. The true requirement for those who obtain their vitamin D solely from diet may be at least 15 mcg (600 IU/day).

"Several factors contribute to the high risk of vitamin D deficiency in seniors," Holick continued. "Elderly people generally do not obtain sufficient vitamin D in their diets to meet their needs. Also, older people have a decreased capacity to produce vitamin D in their skin. When healthy young and elderly volunteers were exposed to the same amount of sunlight, circulating vitamin D concentrations in the older people increased only to a maximum of 8 ng/ml, compared with 30 ng/ml in the younger people."

For most people, casual exposure to sunlight—rather than planned sunbathing or diet—is the most important contributor to the vitamin D requirement,

Holick continued. Many factors, such as seasonal changes, time of day, latitude, sunscreen use, and skin pigmentation can influence the production of vitamin D in the skin.

"Those who do not receive enough vitamin D from sunlight exposure must rely on dietary sources," Holick said. "Because many of the foods sold in Western countries are fortified with vitamins, it is often assumed that vitamin D deficiency should not be a problem. However, the only major food product that is fortified with vitamin D is milk and recent investigations have indicated that the amount of the vitamin in milk samples is substantially lower than the amount on the label. Thus, it may be unwise to recommend milk as the sole source of vitamin D."

Women sixty-five years of age or older should be screened to find out if their bones contain enough calcium and other minerals, according to Isadore Rosenfeld, MD.[6]

"If you are especially vulnerable, that is, you are thin, have a small frame, and a history of fractures, or have a calcium and vitamin D deficiency, you should be tested earlier," he said. "For women at risk, I recommend 1,200 mg/day of calcium citrate and 1,000 IU day of vitamin D."

With an estimated lifetime risk of fractures of more than 40 percent for women and 13 percent for men, osteoporosis is well-recognized as a major public health problem, reported Katherine L. Tucker of Tufts University in Boston and researchers at other facilities. Although a great deal of attention has been given to the importance of calcium and vitamin D, much less is known about the effects of other nutrients contributing to the development of bone, such as potassium, magnesium, vitamin K, and nutrients in fruits and vegetables.[7]

In their study, based on data from the famous Framingham Heart Study, 907 volunteers, who ranged in age from sixty-nine to ninety-three, filled out food questionnaires as part of an osteoporosis study. Six dietary patterns were identified: (1) meat, dairy, and bread; (2) meat and sweet baked products; (3) sweet baked products; (4) alcohol; (5) candy; and (6) fruit, vegetables, and cereal.

After adjusting for variables, men in the last group had significantly greater bone mineral density than did those in two to four of the other groups at the hip sites and the candy group at the radius. Men in the candy group had significantly lower BMD than did those in the fruit, vegetable, and cereal group for three of the four sites. Women in the candy group had significantly lower BMD than did all but one other group in the radius.

"In the present analysis, those with the highest protein intake were in the meat, dairy, and bread, and in the meat and sweet baked products group, both with average BMD that were higher than those of the candy group, but lower than those of the fruit, vegetable, and cereal groups," the researchers added.

These groups also had higher intakes of calcium, vitamin D, phosphorus, magnesium, potassium, and vitamin C than did the alcohol, candy, or sweet baked products groups, the researchers continued. Consistent with these overall nutrient profiles, the candy group, followed by the sweet baked products group, had the lowest bone mineral density, suggesting that the displacement of nutrient-rich bone foods in the diet may explain why high intakes of these foods is detrimental to bone health.

In seniors living independently or in nursing homes, with a mean age of 82.8 years, those who were injected with 150,000 to 300,000 IU of vitamin D_2 once a year for four years showed fewer fractures of all types, compared to the controls who were not given the vitamin, reported *Osteoporosis International.*[8]

Calcitriol (1,25-dihydroxyvitamin D_3) increases gastrointestinal absorption of calcium and stimulates osteoblastic activity in the skeleton, according to researchers at the University of Otago in New Zealand. They added that this is an effective treatment for osteoporosis.[9]

In the three-year, single-blind study, 622 women with one or more vertebral fractures were randomly assigned to take calcitriol (0.25 mcg twice daily) or supplemental calcium at 1 g/day (1,000 mg). Fractures were monitored each year during the study.

The study, reported in the *New England Journal of Medicine,* found that the rate of new vertebral fractures was reduced threefold during the second and third year in the women who took calcitriol, compared to the women only taking calcium. It was also reported that calcitriol was effective in patients with normal calcium absorption and in those with calcium malabsorption. No adverse side effects were recorded.

Exercise intervention in the elderly has been reported to decrease the frequency of falls in 10 percent of the patients, reported Ian R. Reid, MD, of the University of Auckland, New Zealand. Calcium at 1,000 mg/day is adequate in estrogen-replete women, while 1,500 mg/day is probably necessary in postmenopausal women not taking hormone replacement therapy. Calcium supplementation in postmenopausal women produces small but statistically significant benefit on axial bone density in those more than five years after menopause, he added.[10]

He goes on to say that vitamin D deficiency can be treated or prevented with daily use of calciferol at doses on the order of 500–2,000 IU/day or with inter-mittent larger doses up to 100,000 IU/month. Vitamin D therapy has been found to help prevent hip fractures in which calciferol intake was between 0.25 and 0.5 mcg/day, he reported in the *American Journal of the Medical Sciences.*

A reduction of gut calcium absorption may be due to a vitamin D deficien-cy or estrogen deficiency, and vitamin D stimulates calcium absorption in the gut, according to Richard L. Prince, MD, writing in the *New England Journal of Medicine.* When calcium intake is high, passive absorption is necessary. A vita-min D deficiency is commonly found in sunlight-deprived people, but if a vitamin D deficiency is caused by a lack of sunlight exposure, then vitamin D supplementation with ergocalciferol (vitamin D_2) or cholecalciferol (vitamin D_3) will suffice, he said.[11]

If there is a defect in kidney synthesis of 1,25-dihydroxyvitamin D (calcitri-ol), then exogenous calcitriol may be necessary, he added. Supplementation with calcium and vitamin D has brought a reduction of 30–70 percent in fracture rates over two to four years. Evidence suggests that calcium intake must be at least 1,200 mg/day and that sunlight-deprived seniors in nursing homes might require calcium and vitamin D supplements.

Writing in the *New England Journal of Medicine,* Philip Sambrook, MD, of St. Vincent's Hospital in Darlinghurst, New South Wales, Australia, and col-leagues, evaluated the effects of calcium, calcitriol, and calcitonin for the pos-sible prevention of corticosteroid-induced osteoporosis. Corticosteroids (steroids) are used as immunosuppressive agents, as well as anti-inflammatory agents for bone pain, arthritis, and the like.[12]

The study involved 103 patients undergoing corticosteroid therapy who were randomly assigned to take (1) 1,000 mg/day of calcium orally and either cal-citriol at 0.5 to 1.0 mcg/day orally, plus salmon calcitonin at 400 IU/day intra-muscularly, (2) calcitriol plus a placebo nasal spray, or (3) a double placebo for one year.

At the end of the study, data on ninety-two patients had been collected. Bone density was measured by photon absorptiometry every four months for two years. Calcitriol at a mean dose of 0.6 mcg/day, with or without calcitonin, pre-vented more bone loss from the lumbar spine than calcium alone. However, bone loss at the femoral neck and distal radius was not significantly affected by the therapy.

In the second year of the study, lumbar bone loss did not occur in the group previously treated with calcitonin plus calcitriol, but it did in the group given only calcium.

The calcitriol group also lost lumbar bone, but they received more corticosteroids in the second year than the other two groups, the researchers continued. However, they added, calcitriol and calcium used prophylactically, with or without calcitonin, prevent corticosteroid-induced bone loss in the lumbar spine.

Their findings suggest that the prevention of bone loss from the lumbar spine can be achieved with treatment with calcium and calcitriol, with some additional long-term effects possible with calcitonin.

Osteoporosis in men continues to be underdiagnosed and undertreated, according to Peter R. Ebeling, MD, of Royal Melbourne Hospital and Western Hospital in Australia.[13]

For men seventy and older, and younger men with clinical risk factors for osteoporosis, Ebeling said bone density should be measured by dual-energy x-ray absorptiometry. "I would also measure levels of serum total testosterone and 25-hydroxyvitamin D," he added. "A calcium intake of at least 1,200 mg/day, and vitamin D supplementation of at least 800 IU/day, should be recommended, as should regular weight-bearing exercise."

Oral bisphosphonate, considered the first-line treatment for osteoporosis in men, should be recommended, with patient education regarding potential side effects, he said.

20.

Prostate Problems

A solid, chestnut-shaped organ surrounding the first part of the urethra in males, the prostate gland is located under the bladder and in front of the rectum, explained the *American Medical Association Home Medical Encyclopedia.*[1]

The gland produces secretions from part of the seminal fluid during ejaculation. The ejaculatory ducts from the seminal vesicles pass through the prostate to enter the urethra.

"The prostate weighs only a few grams at birth and enlargement begins at puberty due to androgen hormones and it stops growing about the age of 20," the publication said. "At that point, it reaches its adult weight of about 20 grams. In most men, the prostate begins to grow larger after the age of 50."

The gland consists of two main zones: (1) an inner zone, which produces secretions responsible for keeping the lining of the urethra moist; and (2) an outer layer, which produces seminal secretions.

Prostate problems rarely surface before the age of thirty, the publication continued. Prostatitis, an inflammation of the prostate, is often caused by a bacterial infection, which may be sexually transmitted. Enlargement of the prostate (benign prostatic hyperplasia, or BPH) usually affects men over fifty, inhibiting urination by compressing the urethra.

Prostate cancer, which is often a disease of old age, may cause symptoms similar to those caused by an enlarged prostate. Enlargement of the prostate can be detected during a digital rectal exam or through a PSA (prostate-specific antigen) blood test.

Writing in the July 19, 2007, issue of the *New England Journal of Medicine,* Michael F. Holick, MD, PhD, of the Boston University School of Medicine, said that people living in higher altitudes are at an increased risk for prostate, colon, pancreatic, ovarian, breast, Hodgkin's lymphoma, and other cancers, when compared with people living at lower altitudes.[2]

He added that a number of epidemiological studies suggest that levels of 25-hydroxyvitamin D below 20 ng/ml are associated with a 30–50 percent increased risk of prostate, colon, and breast cancer, including a higher mortality from these cancers. For example, in a study of men with prostate cancer, the disease developed three to five years later in men who worked outdoors than in those who worked indoors.

The question here is this: since the kidneys tightly regulate the production of 1,25-dihydroxyvitamin D, why do blood levels not rise in response to an increased exposure to sunlight or increased intake of vitamin D? Holick asked. In addition, in a vitamin D–insufficient state, 1,25-dihydroxyvitamin D levels are often normal or even elevated. The obvious explanation is that prostate, colon, breast, and other tissues express 25-hydroxyvitamin D-1-alphahydroxylase and produce 1,25-dihydroxyvitamin D locally to control genes that help to prevent cancer by keeping cellular proliferation and differentiation in check.

"It has been suggested," Holick added, "that if a cell becomes malignant, 1,25-dihydroxyvitamin D can induce apoptosis [cell death] and prevent angiogenesis [development of new blood vessels], thereby reducing the potential for the malignant cell to survive."

Holick added that once 1,25-dihydroxyvitamin D completes these tasks, it initiates its own destruction by stimulating the CYP24 gene to produce the inactive calcitroic acid. This guarantees that 1,25-dihydroxyvitamin D does not enter the circulation to influence calcium metabolism. This is a plausible explanation for why increased sun exposure and higher circulating levels of 25-hydroxyvitamin D in the blood are associated with a decreased risk of deadly cancers.

When scientists discovered that most tissues and cells in the body have a vitamin D receptor and that several possess the enzymatic machinery to convert the primary circulating form of vitamin D—25-hydroxyvitamin D—to the active form—1,25-dihydroxyvitamin D—this provided new insights into the function of this vitamin, Holick said.

We get vitamin D from sun exposure, from the diet, and from dietary supplements. A diet high in oily fish prevents vitamin D deficiency. Solar UV-B radiation—wavelengths of 290–315 nanometer (nm), one-billionth of a meter—penetrates the skin and converts 7-dehydrocholesterol to previtamin D_3, which is readily converted to vitamin D_3. Since any excess previtamin D_3, or vitamin D_3, is destroyed by sunlight, excessive exposure to sunlight does not cause vitamin D_3 intoxication.

Unfortunately, Holick continued, few foods naturally contain vitamin D or are fortified with it. The *D* in this instance refers to D_2 or D_3. Vitamin D_2 is manufactured through the ultraviolet irradiation of ergosterol from yeast and vitamin D_3 through the UV irradiation of 7-dehydrocholesterol from lanolin. Both are available in over-the-counter vitamin D supplements; however, the form found in prescriptions in the United States is often vitamin D_2. However, D_3 supplements are also available over the counter.

Vitamin D from the skin and diet is metabolized in the liver to 25-hydroxyvitamin D, which is used to determine a patient's vitamin D status, Holick continued. In effect, 25-hydroxyvitamin D is metabolized in the kidneys by the enzyme 25-hydroxyvitamin D-1-alpha-hydroxylase (CYP27B1) to its active form, 1,25-dihydroxyvitamin D. The kidney production of 1,25-dihydroxyvitamin D is tightly regulated by plasma parathyroid hormone levels and blood levels of calcium and phosphorus.

Holick goes on to say that vitamin D intoxication is extremely rare, but it can be caused by inadvertent or intentional ingestion of excessively high doses of the vitamin. Doses over 50,000 IU/day can raise levels of 25-hydroxyvitamin D to more than 150 ng/ml, resulting in hypercalcemia and hyperphosphatemia; that is, elevated levels of calcium and phosphorus. Doses of 10,000 IU/day of vitamin D_3 for up to five months do not cause toxicity.

"Much evidence suggests that the recommended adequate intakes of vitamin D are actually inadequate and need to be increased to at least 800 IU/day of vitamin D_3," Holick said. "However, unless a person eats oily fish frequently, it is very difficult to obtain that much vitamin D_3 on a daily basis from dietary sources. Excessive exposure to sunlight, especially sunlight that causes sunburn, will increase the risk of skin cancer. Thus, sensible sun exposure—or UV-B irradiation—and the use of supplements are needed to fulfill the body's vitamin D requirements."

At the Orentreich Foundation for the Advancement of Science in Cold Spring-on-the-Hudson, New York, Joseph H. Vogelman and colleagues evaluated 181 cases of prostate cancer, which included 90 African Americans and 91 whites.[3]

The research team reported that those with elevated risks of prostate cancer had lower summer levels of 1,25-dihydroxyvitamin D. This suggests that the conversion of 25-hydroxyvitamin D to 1,25-dihydroxyvitamin D affects the risk of prostate cancer.

Patients would be expected to have more vitamin D available in the body in the summer, since the sun can interact with hormones in the skin to produce the vitamin, the researchers added.

Accepted risk factors for prostate cancer are age and race/ethnicity, in which African American men have the highest prostate cancer risk in the world, while Japanese and Chinese men native to those countries have the lowest rates, reported the *Journal of the National Cancer Institute.*[4]

There is a strong familial risk that has been related to genetics, and there appears to be a strong inverse relationship between circulating blood levels of 1,25-dihydroxyvitamin D and prostate cancer development, according to Ronald K. Ross, MD, of the University of Southern California/Norris Comprehensive Cancer Center in Los Angeles.

As reported in *Cancer Research,* men who have a particular type of vitamin D receptor gene are more likely than others to develop prostate cancer. In studying 108 cancer patients undergoing surgical removal of the prostate, compared with 170 men who did not have prostate cancer, the men with the cancer were more likely to carry two copies of a recessive vitamin D–receptor gene.[5]

Cancerous prostate cells are vulnerable to vitamin D_3, making the vitamin good for both prevention and treatment, reported Robert C. Atkins, MD. The only downside is that rather large amounts are necessary, which may raise the body's calcium level precipitously. The vitamin stops tumor cells from spreading, and it has reduced cancerous growths by over 50 percent, he added.[6]

Mortality rates from multiple sclerosis (MS) show a well-known north–south gradient, similar to prostate cancer internationally and in the United States, according to Gary G. Schwartz, PhD, of the University of Pittsburgh School of Medicine.[7]

Prostate cancer has been added to a list of diseases whose geographical distribution is significantly correlated with multiple sclerosis. These include colon cancer, dental caries, and Parkinson's disease, and these diseases may share an aberration in vitamin D metabolism.

Evidence demonstrating a multifaceted role for vitamin D in immunoregulation suggests that a vitamin D aberration may contribute to the etiology of multiple sclerosis. The pathogenesis of MS is related to T-cell-mediated events, Schwartz added.

Advances in the immunobiology of vitamin D suggests this hypothesis for the etiology of MS. Multiple sclerosis results from an inflammatory response triggered by exogenous (outside the body) factors, such as viral infections, trauma, or lesions in the central nervous system in genetically susceptible people.

Low levels of biologically active vitamin D may fail to inhibit the inflammatory T-cell response, Schwartz continued. These activated T-cells interact with neural (nerve) tissue, which results in sensitization against neural antigens, or what is referred to as *autoimmunization.* The latter can result in chronic neurologic disease.

Dark-skinned African American men, who have the highest incidence of prostate cancer, absorb less sunlight and, therefore, have lower levels of vitamin D than do fair-skinned men, according to Peter T. Scardino, MD. With age, the body's ability to manufacture vitamin D diminishes and the incidence of prostate cancer increases.[8]

Vitamin D regulates gene expression and modulates cellular proliferation and differentiation, according to D. M. Peehl of Stanford University School of Medicine in Palo Alto, California, and colleagues. In a lab test, normal BPH and malignant tissues were evaluated for their response to $1,25(OH)_2D_3$, and it was found that the growth of epithelial strains derived from the normal, benign, prostatic, and cancer tissues was inhibited by vitamin D.[9]

Stromal cells—connective tissue—appear to be less sensitive to vitamin D, but growth inhibition of epithelial cells by the vitamin was irreversible. Even limited exposure of less than two hours to vitamin D severely inhibited the cells' ability to proliferate after removal of the hormone/vitamin.

It was found that vitamin D did not alter the morphology (structural form) or alter epithelial cell expression of keratins (epidermal tissue) associated with either secretory or squamous differentiation. While vitamin D irreversibly inhibited growth, it did not appear to do so by the induction of apoptosis (death of a cell) or differentiation. Vitamin D seems to put cells into a type of permanent nonproliferative state. Also, vitamin D inhibited cells from generating possible adenocarcinomas (glandular cancer), Peehl added.

Men with prostate cancer have lower blood levels of the hormonal form of vitamin D—1,25-dihydroxyvitamin D—according to a study reported in *Family Practice News.* This hormonal form seems to maintain differentiation of prostate cells.[10]

Mortality rates from prostate cancer are invariably correlated with the availability of ultraviolet radiation, the principal source of vitamin D. Sunlight and vitamin D products may also be protective against colon, rectum, breast, and ovarian cancer.

Studies have shown an incidence of malignancy six to ten times lower in latitudes closer to the equator, in those who receive more sunlight. Sunlight may also protect against melanoma, although this skin cancer incidence is not necessarily proportional to cumulative sun exposure.

Several studies have indicated there is a pathophysiological relationship between rather high levels of calcium in the blood, which could promote prostate cancer by reducing the production of vitamin D (1,25(OH)$_2$D), the hormonal form of vitamin D.[11]

However, as reported in the *British Journal of Nutrition* in 2007, changes in blood levels of vitamin D in response to calcium intake are of very small magnitude when compared with the variations required to influence the proliferation and differentiation of prostate cancer cells. In fact, most studies show that vitamin D levels were not found to be reduced in prostate cancer patients.

The researchers added that a recent randomized, placebo-controlled trial did not indicate that calcium supplementation increases the risk of prostate cancer.

The research team added that a link between relatively high calcium intake and consequent low production and circulating blood levels of vitamin D, which might promote prostate cancer, remains a hypothesis, the plausibility of which is not supported by available clinical data.

21.

Rickets

In the first century A.D., Soramus of Ephesus, a Greek gynecologist, obstetrician, and pediatrician, gave a full description of rickets in Roman children as part of his treatise on the diseases of women, reported the *Foods & Nutrition Encyclopedia*. He theorized that this softening and deformation of the bones was caused by children who sat indoors or on damp floors.[1]

The initial report of the disease in Britain was published in 1645, in a doctor of medicine thesis of Dr. Whistler at Oxford University. When the Industrial Revolution was well under way in the nineteenth century, rickets was widespread, as urban residents lived under clouds of black smoke from the burning of soft coal, meaning that the ultraviolet rays of the sun were largely screened out and were insufficient to produce vitamin D.

However, Whistler's thesis was not as widely circulated as was the 1650 account of the disease by Dr. Glissin, a London physician. This report gave the clinical signs of rickets when it occurred by itself and when it was complicated by the existence of scurvy, the vitamin C–codeficient disease.

"An understanding of rickets, however, required the development of better chemical methods for the analysis of bone," the publication said. An accurate analysis of the proportion of calcium and phosphorus in bone was reported by Baron Jons Jakob Berzelius (1779–1848), the Swedish chemist, in 1801.

Details of bone were enhanced by two major German publications in 1858, when Dr. Muller gave a lengthy description of bone growth and the healing process of rickets, while Dr. Pommer described, in detail, features of rickets, osteomalacia, and osteoporosis.

Cod-liver oil was used extensively in the nineteenth century in England to treat tuberculosis and rickets, even though physicians were unsure of its value. These doubts were dispelled in 1889 by a report from the British physician Dr.

Bland-Sutton, who cured the deformed bones of animals at the London zoo by feeding them supplements of crushed bones and cod-liver oil, the publication added.

Only in recent years have people around the world relied on foods such as cod-liver oil and liver as sources of vitamin D. However, it is reported that taking cod-liver oil as a prophylactic remedy by Norwegian fishermen and sailors goes back to the Vikings in the eighth and ninth centuries.

"The addition of vitamin D to fluid whole milk—thereby resulting in a widely used food providing calcium, phosphorus, and vitamin D—has been credited with the virtual elimination of rickets among children in the United States," the publication continued. "The vitamin D fortification of milk to provide a concentration of 400 IU/quart has been endorsed by the Food and Nutrition Board, Nutritional Research Council/National Academy of Sciences, the American Academy of Pediatrics, and the American Medical Association."

A five-month-old boy who had dilated cardiomyopathy (disease of the heart muscle) was found to have hypocalcemia due to vitamin D–deficiency rickets, reported the *Canadian Journal of Cardiology.* Supplementation with calcitriol at 0.15 mg twice daily; calcium gluconate at 250 mg twice daily; elemental calcium twice daily; and magnesium at 50 mg three times daily; with the eventual change of calcitriol to vitamin D_3 at 4,000 IU/day orally, resulted in a resolution of the cardiomyopathy following six months of therapy.[2]

At the Medical College of Georgia in Augusta, Joseph H. Clark, MD, and colleagues, evaluated an eight-year-old boy who developed a limp and a swelling in the fibrous membrane covering the bone. He was found to be hypocalcemic—low levels of calcium in the blood—and there was radiographic evidence of rickets.[3]

It was also found that his vitamin A level was undetectable and his vitamin D readings were low. His diet for several years had consisted of nothing but french fried potatoes and water.

There was considerable improvement in his condition with appropriate supplementation of dihydrotachysterol (now replaced by calcitriol and its derivatives) at 0.25 mg twice daily; 50 mg/kg of elemental calcium daily; and 50,000 IU/day of vitamin A for seven days. The vitamin A supplement was decreased to 5,000 IU/day, and serum vitamin A and retinol-binding protein concentrations remained normal.

Following ten weeks of therapy, ophthalmological examination was entirely normal and his total and ionized calcium normalized within several days.

Within ten weeks, his rickets healed radiographically and, after two months, all supplements were discontinued.

The boy refused food, in spite of three months of intensive psychotherapy, and he was eventually discharged to a chronic care facility, where he was given 40 ounces (1,134g)/day of nasogastric Pediasure. (While there is a smidgen of calcium in french fries, there is no vitamin D.)

An estimated 20–34 percent of Asian toddlers in Great Britain are deficient in vitamin D, and they may also have low iron stores in their blood, according to B. A. Wharton of the Institute of Child Health in London. This puts the children at risk for rickets and anemia, reported the *British Medical Journal*.[4]

Wharton suggested that all pregnant women, and children up to the age of five, should be given a vitamin D supplement, unless they are getting sufficient amounts of the vitamin from the sun and their diet.

A single dose of vitamin D at 600,000 IU or 15,000 mcg of the vitamin, given orally in doses of 100,000 IU every two hours for a twelve-hour period, was given to forty-two patients with rickets, reported the *Journal of Pediatrics*. This therapy, called Stoss Therapy, is safe and effective and eliminates the problem of compliance, according to Binita R. Shah, MD.[5]

This therapy also evokes a response in four to seven days in nutritional rickets, and it becomes a valuable diagnostic aid for patients in whom the initial findings do not clearly distinguish rickets from familial hypophosphatemic (low amounts of phosphorus) rickets, Shah said.

In the study, conducted at Children's Medical Center in Brooklyn, 50,000 IU capsules of ergocalciferol were softened by presoaking them in a small amount of water and the intact capsules were then given in food.

The diagnosis of nutritional rickets is confirmed by low blood levels of calcidiol, which accurately reflects the vitamin D status of the body, Shah added. The large deposit of vitamin D by the Stoss Therapy not only cures rickets, but normal calcidiol levels are also maintained for up to about three months.

Calcidiol (25-hydroxycholecalciferol) is the first step in the conversion of vitamin D_3 to the more active form—calcitriol. It is more potent than vitamin D_3.

In spite of ample sunshine in Saudi Arabia, 1.8 percent of pediatric admissions to the hospital in Riyadh are related to rickets, reported Gulam Nabi, MD, in the *Annals of Saudi Medicine*. However, this disease is uncommon in the southern part of the country at the Khamis Mushayt, which is 7,000 feet (2,134m) above sea level.[6]

Rickets constitutes 0.08 percent of the total admissions to pediatric wards and 0.16 percent of the consultations at outpatient clinics attended in the author's hospital. This low incidence may be explained by the following factors: (1) children enjoy enough sunshine because of the pleasant weather throughout the year; and (2) bottle feeding, which contains supplemental vitamin D, which is common along with breastfeeding. At six months of age, 50 percent of the children are bottle-fed.

Respiratory infection is a major complication of rickets, and Nabi suggests that rickets in Riyadh is a multifactorial problem, in which health education is the key.

Replying to Dr. Nabi's article, Hussein Salman, MD, of Suleimania Children's Hospital in Riyadh, said that rickets, in spite of the sunshine, may be due to the following factors: (1) prolonged breastfeeding without adequate diversification; (2) traditional avoidance of sun exposure; (3) clothing styles; (4) rapid urbanization and housing design with small windows; (5) maternal vitamin D deficiency; and (6) low vitamin D status in the Saudi population, especially in women. The author urged vitamin D supplementation.[7]

22.

Skin Disorders

The largest organ of the body, the skin provides the body surface with a protective coating. It is also an important sensory organ that detects such external conditions as heat and cold. Through the sensation of pain, nerves in the skin notify the brain of any injury to the body, reported *The Book of Health.*[1]

"The skin of an adult normally weighs from six to seven and one-half pounds (2.7–3.4kg) or about twice the weight of the liver," the publication said. "It has a surface area of about 2 square yards (0.5m^2). In thickness, it varies from one thirty-second to one-eighth inch (0.8–3mm)."

The skin is composed of several layers of specialized skin, along with numerous glands, nerves, hairs, hair follicles, and blood vessels. The outer portion of the skin is called the epidermis. This represents only a small portion of the thickness of the skin, and normally, it contains no blood vessels or nerves. The outer layer is called the cornfield layer, or the stratum corneum, which contains the dead cells that are constantly being sloughed off. It is tough because it contains a hornlike material called keratin. The outer layer also contains a large amount of fatty material.

There is a second and lighter layer of the skin, the stratum lucidum, which is located directly below the horny layer of the epidermis, and it is especially prominent on the palms and the soles of the feet.

"The innermost layer of the epidermis, the stratum mucosum, contains most of the melanin pigment of the skin," the publication continued. "The dermis is the layer of the skin which lies just below the epidermis. Most of the structures from which the hairs grow (hair follicles) are located in this layer."

The third major layer of the skin is located below the dermis. It is called the subdermis and it contains mostly fatty tissue. This layer is responsible for most of the insulating ability of the skin, and it varies in depth.

Since the skin covers such a large area of the body, it is subjected to a variety of skin problems, of which sunburn is just one example.

PSORIASIS

The continuous loss of worn cells from the skin's surface balances the continuous production of new cells in the basal layer of the epidermis, explained *The Physicians' Manual for Patients*.[2]

A healthy cell passes from the basal layer to the surface in about two months, during which time it gradually forms an accumulation of keratin. However, for some reasons not completely understood, in psoriasis there is an abnormally fast rate of cell production. In effect, the new cells reach the surface in as little as six days and do not have time to accumulate keratin. This results in the unsightly flaking of the skin in psoriasis.

"Psoriasis is a fairly common condition," the publication said. "For example, 2 to 4 percent of white Americans—far fewer blacks—suffer from this disorder in varying degrees of intensity. While it is unusual before puberty, thereafter it can appear for the first time at any age. Almost 30 percent of those with psoriasis have a family history of the disease."

Psoriasis and arthritis sometimes appear together. Psoriasis is a long-term condition because it flares up unpredictably and then subsides—perhaps for years—but it never clears up completely without intervention. However, it is not contagious.

Psoriasis usually begins as small red spots and white scales. The lesions can be itchy or sore. As the disease progresses, the small areas may merge or form bright red patches covered with scales that resemble mica, or the inside of an oyster shell. The patches can grow progressively larger and blend together, the publication continued.

"In one form, known as exfoliative psoriatic dermatitis, the skin is red and covered with fine scales that often obscure the typical lesions. Scarring pustules, usually on the palms of the hands and the soles of the feet, are characteristic of another form called pustular psoriasis," the publication said.

The most common sites of psoriasis are the scalp—usually behind the ears—the knees, the elbows, the back, and the buttocks. Less frequently, patches are found on the hands, under the breasts, in the genital area, or in the armpits. In some cases, the nails are affected, becoming thick and pitted, but the face is usually spared.

"Many factors can trigger psoriasis, including stress, allergies, severe sunburn, throat infections, and exposure to excessive cold," the publication added. "Often a surgical incision or a cut or burn precipitates an eruption at the site of the wound. Sometimes localized psoriasis appears at pressure points—on the hands of mail carriers and golfers. Once the condition has been established, it persists even when the triggering factor ceases."

As reported in the *British Journal of Dermatology,* vitamin D and its analogs are beneficial in the treatment of psoriasis. Possible adverse complications include interference with endogenous (inside the body) vitamin D metabolism, altered intestinal absorption of calcium and phosphate, an effect on the mineralization of bone, and an effect on PCTH reduction. Examples of synthetic vitamin D analogs are calcipotriol, calcitriol, and tacalcitol.[3]

As explained by J. F. Bourke and colleagues at the Leicester Royal Infirmary in Great Britain, vitamin D_3 is made from provitamin D_3 that is exposed to UV-B radiation through the skin. Vitamin D_3 is then converted to 25-hydroxyvitamin D_3. In the kidneys, vitamin D is then converted in the liver to calcitriol, which increases the absorption of calcium and phosphorus in the small intestine.

Bourke goes on to say that moderately extensive chronic plaque psoriasis responds to approximately 100 g/week of calcipotriol at a concentration of 50 mcg/g.

In seven patients with psoriasis vulgaris, a clinical trial of topical vitamin D_3 showed that four of the seven patients experienced complete remission and marked improvement and two others reported minimal improvement of their skin lesions during the treatment period, according to *Calcified Tissue International.* No adverse reactions were reported.[4]

In another issue of the same journal, five volunteers with persistent psoriasis were given 1,25-dihydroxyvitamin D topically at 0.1 mcg/g and 0.2 mcg/g. Results indicated a definite and sometimes remarkable improvement in skin lesions at the concentration of 0.5 mcg/g when applied for two to five weeks. No toxicity was reported.[5]

Low blood levels of vitamin D have been associated with psoriasis, especially in postular varieties, according to Luigi Naldi, MD, of Università degli Studi di Milano in Bergamo, Italy.[6]

Topically applied vitamin D derivatives are effective in relieving the symptoms of established psoriasis, Naldi reported in the *British Journal of Dermatology.* In addition, retinoids (vitamin A) are well-established systemic treatments for severe psoriasis. The amount of calories ingested may also play a role.

In another article in the just-cited journal, 3 mcg/g of 1,25-dihydroxyvitamin

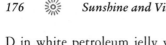

D in white petroleum jelly was given topically to ten patients with psoriasis. There was a statistically significant reduction of psoriasis inflammation and epidermal proliferation and keratinization with the vitamin D therapy, the researchers said.[7]

According to an article in the *Journal of Dermatological Science,* the vitamin D receptor VDR and the gene that converts this receptor regulate the levels of vitamin D in the body. As reported in this study, patients with psoriasis had structural polymorphisms (an occurrence in more than one form) in their VDR gene, which resulted in impairments in the receptor binding and metabolism of the vitamin. This discovery suggests that defective metabolism of vitamin D may predispose people to psoriasis.[8]

As reported in the *British Journal of Dermatology,* eighty-five patients with psoriasis that involved 15 percent of their body surface were asked to ingest no more than 800 mg/day of calcium from their diet for twenty-four hours and they were placed on 0.5 mcg of calcitriol (1,25-dihydroxyvitamin D_3) at bedtime. The vitamin D was increased in increments of 0.05 mcg every two weeks to an average of 2.4 mcg/day, with some patients taking 4.0 mcg at night.[9]

It was found that 88 percent had some improvement in their condition under this regimen. The psoriasis area of severity index score was reduced after six and twenty-four months on the oral vitamin D therapy. Blood calcium concentrations and twenty-four-hour urinary calcium excretion increased 3.9 and 148.2 percent, respectively, but they were not outside the normal range. Following six months of oral vitamin D, there was a 22.5 percent decline in creatinine clearance. The researchers added that oral calcitriol is an effective and safe treatment for psoriasis. Creatinine is a component of urine excretion.

Topical vitamin D analogs are a new, effective, more convenient, and better-tolerated option for the treatment of psoriasis, according to an article by J. Barth-Jones and P. H. Hutchinson of Leicester Royal Infirmary in Great Britain.[10]

Psoriasis vulgaris is the major form of this disease studied with vitamin D antagonists, and both calcitriol and calcipotriol have been shown to be effective in numerous clinical trials, they said. Calcipotriol has compared well with betamethasone valerate and short-contact dithranol in controlled studies.

These vitamin D analogs appear to directly affect the regulation of keratinocyte proliferation and differentiation, the researchers added. These compounds also have potent immunological properties, and they may act by inhibiting cytokine production by keratinocytes or lymphocytes.

Topical applications of these nutrients appear to be safe, but hypercalcemia and hypercalcuria may develop if large quantities are used. Oral calcitriol has been used at 0.25 to 0.5 mcg/day and topically from 3 to 15 mcg/g.

Calcipotriol has been the vitamin D analog used most extensively in the treatment of psoriasis, according to K. Kragballe, MD, of the University of Aarhus in Denmark. Compared with $1,25(OH)_2D_2$, calcipotriol is about two hundred times less potent in its effect on calcium metabolism, although it has a similar receptor affinity.[11]

Topically applied at 50 mcg/g twice daily, it is safe and effective for the treatment of psoriasis. It's slightly more effective than betamethasone, Kragballe said, and the doctor feels that it should be the first drug of choice in the management of psoriasis.

Kragballe added that the rationale for the use of vitamin D analogs in the treatment of psoriasis is to reverse the epidermal hyperproliferation and promote epidermal differentiation. Vitamin D analogs also possess immunosuppressive properties, and the researchers have wondered if immunosuppression is not what causes the antipsoriatic effect.

As reported in *Hautarzt,* 1,25-dihydroxyvitamin D_3 was discovered to be a member of the nuclear steroid hormone receptor family. This family of the gene regulating DNA-binding proteins includes the estrogen, progesterone, glucocorticoid, mineral corticoid, thyroxine, and tetinoic acid receptors.[12]

In fact, vitamin D receptors have been identified in a variety of tissues primarily unrelated to calcium metabolism, according to Petra Milde, MD, of Hautklink der Heinrich-Heine Universitat in Düsseldorf, Germany.

The skin and the immune system, both involved in psoriasis, are some of the most interesting new targets, she added. In vitro, 1,25-dihydroxyvitamin D_3 inhibits proliferation and induces differentiation of keratinocytes, and this vitamin/hormone has potent immune-modulating functions. *Differentiation* essentially means a different diagnosis, that is, the acquisition of characteristics different from that of the original type.

SCLERODERMA

This disease, also known as progressive systemic sclerosis, is a disorder characterized by an excessive buildup of fibrous connective tissue, according to the *Columbia University College of Physicians and Surgeons Complete Home Medical Guide.* *Scleroderma* means thickening (sclero) of the skin (derma) and it was initially thought to involve the skin alone. However, vital internal organs may also be targets of increased collagen deposits. Hence, the term *progressive systemic sclerosis* (PSS).[13]

"In PSS, there is often an associated arthritis, even though the joints are not the main targets of the disease," the publication said. "In addition to mild joint inflammation, there are changes in the tissues around the joints because of deposition of excessive amounts of connective tissue. This results in reduced mobility. With the progressive thickening and tightness of the skin about the fingers, motion becomes increasingly restricted. Elbows and knees may also be involved."

For reasons not completely understood, the disease seems to be confined to the fibroblasts, the cells that make fibrous connective tissue or collagen. In scleroderma, the fibroblasts behave almost as though they were continually being stimulated to produce collagen. As an example, when we cut ourselves, the wound heals with new connective tissue. Once the cut has healed, the reparative process stops and new collagen ceases to be produced.

In scleroderma, however, fibrous tissue is produced at an accelerated rate, even without the stimulus of a wound, the publication continued. As a result, increasing amounts of new or immature collagen are continuously being laid down in the involved tissues, replacing the normal cells with connective tissue, as though they were a scar. This makes the skin thick and tight, as the normal elastic tissue is replaced by dense fibrous tissue. Hair growth and sweating usually stop because the hair follicles and sweat glands are destroyed in the process.

If the hands are involved, a tightening of the skin over the fingers results in a physical narrowing of the tiny blood vessels necessary for their nourishment, resulting in skin ulceration on the fingertips and joints, and bony protuberances.

"When PSS attacks internal organs, the disease can be life threatening," the publication said. "In the lungs, the disease may cause an increase in connective tissue in the air sacs, a condition called pulmonary fibrosis. Oxygen transfer from the inhaled air to the blood is progressively blocked; blood is deprived of its normal oxygen, leading to a shortness of breath."

If the heart is involved, there may be a replacement of the pericardium, the membrane surrounding the heart, by increased fibrous tissue. More commonly, the heart muscle fibers are replaced with ineffective scar tissue, which leads to heart failure, the publication added.

"In the gastrointestinal tract, PSS may cause difficulty in swallowing, malabsorption of digested food into the circulation or severe constipation and possible intestinal obstruction," the publication continued. "The kidney is another vital organ where PSS may strike, leading to a very severe form of high blood pressure."

Raynaud's syndrome, a condition in which there is blanching of the skin of the hands and feet due to cold exposure, may be associated with PSS, along with lupus, rheumatoid arthritis, and other forms of connective tissue disease.

Many doctors treat scleroderma with drugs that suppress the immune system and reduce inflammation, and nutrition isn't thought to play much of a role in the development and progression of the disease, said Sheldon Paul Blau, MD, of the State University of New York at Stony Brook. But nutrition does play an important role in managing the best possible health despite the disease, he added.[14]

"Most doctors who offer nutritional therapy to their patients with scleroderma are helping them to absorb nutrients more equally by recommending liquid and intravenous feedings and supplements," Blau continued. "Some doctors further suggest dietary changes and add nutrients that are thought to help reduce inflammation and stress on organs such as the heart and kidneys."

He goes on to say that inflammation produces unstable molecules, called *free radicals,* which damage a cell by grabbing electrons from healthy molecules in the cell's outer membrane. Antioxidants offer free radicals their own electrons, thereby disarming the free radicals and saving cells from harm.

Even scleroderma patients who don't require special feeding formulas can benefit from taking a multivitamin/mineral supplement, Blau said. These patients have an especially hard time absorbing the fat-soluble vitamins—A, D, E, and K—and they can develop many symptoms associated with deficiencies of these nutrients if they do not get adequate amounts of them. He has seen patients with scleroderma who developed softened bones from lack of vitamin D and hemorrhaging from a lack of vitamin K.

For two years, a thirty-five-year-old woman with localized scleroderma was given 1,25-dihydroxyvitamin D_3 orally for six months. The researchers reported a beneficial response to the vitamin D therapy during the next six months. It is said that the vitamin may have both immunoregulatory and inhibitory effects on fibroblast growth. Fibroblasts are cells capable of forming collagen fibers.[15]

In a Scandinavian study involving one male and ten females with scleroderma, with a mean age of forty-six, the patients were given 1,25-dihydroxyvitamin D in an oral dose of 1.75 mcg/day. After a treatment period of six months to three years, there was a significant improvement when compared to their status at the beginning of the study. No serious side effects were reported.[16]

In the *Journal of Rheumatology,* researchers evaluated six women and two men, ranging in age from thirty-four to fifty-two, with skin lesions ranging from 7 to 90 percent of their body and with a disease duration of two to sixteen years. They were compared with eight controls who were between thirty-two and forty-seven years of age.[17]

Whole body irradiation with UV-B light showed no significant differences in basal serum vitamin D_3 levels or post–UV-B blood values, although the increases in post–UV-B vitamin D_3 levels were significant in both groups.

In another group of nineteen patients with progressive systemic sclerosis, compared with matched controls, random levels of active vitamin D metabolites, 25-hydroxyvitamin D and 1,25-dihydroxyvitamin D, were similar in both groups. Vitamin D metabolites appear to function normally with patients with progressive systemic sclerosis.

PRURIGO

Prurigo is a chronic disease of the skin that is marked by persistent eruption of papules with constant itching. It can be complicated by systemic diseases, such as lymphoproliferative or metabolic disorders, and it is often accompanied by atopic dermatitis, according to researchers at the Tokyo Medical and Clinical Dental University School of Medicine in Japan.[18]

In eleven patients treated with topical vitamin D_3 ointment (tacalcitol), who had been topical steroid ointment–resistant, nine of the eleven patients showed significant clinical response to the regimen within four weeks. The researchers concluded that vitamin D_3 ointment may be an alternative therapy for steroid-resistant prurigo.

HAILEY-HAILEY DISEASE

Discovered by Hugh E. Hailey, an American dermatologist, Hailey-Hailey disease is a complicated skin condition. It was jointly discovered by W. Howard Hailey (1898–1967), also an American dermatologist, hence the double name. It is also referred to as benign familial chronic pemphigus.[19]

As reported in the *British Journal of Dermatology,* a sixty-five-year-old man had lesions in the axillary and inguinal areas bilaterally (meaning, on two sides). He was treated with a vitamin D ointment (tacalcitol) at 2 mg/g, which resulted in the lesions disappearing in both groin areas, and remission had continued at the time the article was written.

23.

Sunscreens and Vitamin D

Writing in the September 28, 2005, issue of the *Journal of the American Medical Association,* June K. Robinson, MD, editor of *Archives of Dermatology,* referred to an article in her publication in which Elisabeth Thieden and colleagues measured ultraviolet exposure in conjunction with sunscreen use.[1, 2]

While controlled epidemiological studies have shown protective effects from sunscreen use, other epidemiological studies of sunscreen use show increased skin cancer risk associated with the use of sunscreens, Robinson said. One explanation is that sunscreen use is sometimes a marker for those receiving larger short-wave UV doses that are not completely compensated for by the protective effect of sunscreen.

She referred to a study by A. Dupuy and colleagues,[3] which examined the effect of sunscreen at French vacation sites. It was found that those who used SPF 12 sunscreen, as opposed to SPF 40, and experienced redness tended to use more sunscreen. Although sunscreens are not the preferred choice for sun protection—avoidance of the sun and protective clothing that shields the wearer from the sun are the best choices—recommending a high SPF sunscreen is sound advice.

Robinson goes on to say that daily sun exposure is adequate for vitamin D production to occur in fair-skinned people. For example, exposing 5 percent of the skin in fair-skinned people two to three times a week for five minutes of noontime summer sun exposure is equivalent to an intake of 430 IU/day of vitamin D.

"Nonetheless," she added, "vitamin D deficiency does exist in healthy adolescents and it has been reported in the winter months in both younger and older adults. For those fifty-one to seventy, the recommended vitamin D intake is 400 IU/day and 600 IU/day for those older than seventy."

While there is evidence that many people—older and darker-skinned people, in particular—may have low blood levels of vitamin D, increasing exposure to natural or artificial UV light is not recommended as a supplemental source of vitamin D, she said.

"Vitamin D levels are lower in the elderly than in younger people, perhaps due to their thin epidermis having less 7-dehydrocholesterol, the source for the generation of vitamin D by suberythemal UV doses," she continued. "The melanin pigment of the epidermis of darker-skinned people absorbs the UV photons responsible for the photochemical reactions producing previtamin D. Photosynthesizing vitamin D through natural sunlight is maximized after 20 minutes of UV-B exposure. Extended sun exposure provides no additional benefit, but it does increase the likelihood of skin cancer or eye damage."

A multivitamin supplement usually contains 400 IU of vitamin D per tablet, and in the United States, milk is supplemented and contains about 100 IU of vitamin D per eight-ounce glass. A multivitamin tablet taken with a glass of milk provides 500 IU of the vitamin, which meets the current RDA for those younger than seventy; however, some researchers suggest that these recommendations may fail to bring most people up to the desired blood levels of 80 nmol/l, she added.

This is especially true for those who are lactose-intolerant—that is, those who do not secrete the enzyme lactase to deal with the lactose in milk—and consume less milk, so they may need to take nutritional supplements of vitamin D and eat foods rich in the vitamin, such as salmon, mackerel, and the like.

"The recent increasing incidence of skin cancer, especially melanoma, is a cause for concern," Robinson said. "Current estimates are that 1 in 5 people living in the United States will develop skin cancer during their lifetime. In 2005, it is estimated that 105,750 melanomas will be diagnosed in the U.S., that is, 59,580 with invasive melanomas and 46,170 cases of melanoma in situ. And melanomas will claim about 7,770 lives in 2005."

She added that one in four people who develop melanoma is younger than forty and that person's death affects the lives of his or her younger children. The direct cost of treating melanoma will exceed $563 million, with most of the expense attributed to treating the disease in its advanced stages.

Responding to Robinson's article in the March 1, 2006, issue of the *Journal of the American Medical Association,* James Grote, MD, of Pittsfield, Illinois, said that, while the article provided insight into behavioral patterns and concern for the increasing incidence of skin cancer, it did not convey the scope of vitamin

D deficiency in developed countries, the widespread lack of knowledge about this problem in the health care community, or the need for more investigation about this basic human need.[4]

"Vitamin D deficiency remains poorly defined and current estimated estimates are that older people typically require at least 1,300 IU/day of cholecalciferol and that traditional recommendations are inadequate for all ages," Grote said. "Supplemental guidelines for vitamin D were increased earlier this year to 1,000 IU/day for those older than seventy years. Numerous questions remain unanswered, not just about optional dosing, but also about the effects of vitamin D on multiple organ systems."

Very little UV-B radiation reaches the earth above 37 degrees of latitude from November through February, so people who live north of the 37th parallel produce little, if any, vitamin D during late fall and winter, reported Jane Higdon, PhD, in the Linus Pauling Institute Research Report from Oregon State University in Corvallis. She showed a map indicating this meant that part of the United States north of Texas.[5]

"The application of sunscreen with an SPF factor of 8 reduces skin production of vitamin D by 95 percent, even in summer," she added. "The ability to synthesize vitamin D in the skin also decreases with age. A seventy year old makes only 25 percent of the vitamin D made by a twenty year old exposed to the same amount of sunlight."

She reported that exposure of bare arms and legs to sunlight for five to ten minutes two to three times a week improves vitamin D status with minimal risk of skin damage.

An often-asked question is whether or not sunscreens inhibit the formation of vitamin D from the sun. In evaluating vitamin D levels and the use of sunscreens in more than 113 people forty years of age or over, Robin Marks, MPH, and colleagues at the University of Melbourne in Victoria, Australia, reported that over an Australian summer, sufficient sunlight is received, probably through both the sunscreen and the lack of total skin coverage. This provides adequate vitamin D production in those who use sunscreens, Marks said.[6]

The use of sunscreen will diminish the cutaneous synthesis of vitamin D, according to Michael F. Holick, MD, PhD, of Boston University Medical Center in Massachusetts. The elderly are especially at risk for this, he said.[7]

Exposure of the hands, face, and forearms to suberythemal amounts of sunlight two to three times a week ensures adequate vitamin D, he added. If people remain outdoors longer, a sunscreen with a sun protection factor of 15 is recommended. In an Australian population, using sunscreen with a sun protection factor of 17 applied daily to the head and neck, forearms, and dorsal aspects of the hands did not lower vitamin D levels.

There has been a steep rise in the rates of melanoma since the mid-1970s and sun avoidance and the use of chemical sunscreens are the major strategies for risk reduction, explained Cedric F. Garland, Dr. PH, of the University of California at San Diego. However, since the 1970s and 1980s, there has been a continued increase in mortality from melanoma, even with the wide use of high-protectant sunscreens.[8]

Most sunscreens block UV-B radiation, but they do not block UV-A radiation, which is about 90–95 percent of the ultraviolet energy in the solar system, he said. It has been suggested that sunscreens prevent the redness and sunburn effect and, therefore, people using sunscreens are more likely to get excessive exposure of the skin to parts of the solar spectrum other than UV-B radiation.

The researchers believe there is laboratory data supporting the concept that melanoma and basal cell cancers are initiated or promoted by solar radiation other than UV-B. If this is true, then UV-B sunscreens may not only be ineffective in preventing cancers, but the ointments may actually increase a person's risk.

The traditional ways of limiting sun exposure are wearing hats, wearing adequate protective clothing, and avoiding prolonged sunbathing. These suggestions may be more beneficial than relying on sunscreens, the researchers continued.

Chemical sunscreens became popular in the 1960s, and they utilized formulations with low sun protection factors to enhance tanning. Eventually, sunscreens became regarded as chemopreventive agents for skin cancers and the sun protection factors increased.

The researchers added that the age-adjusted incidence and mortality rates from melanoma have actually increased since sunscreens were introduced in Australia. The use of sunscreens has been promoted in Britain, France, Switzerland, and the Scandinavian countries since the 1960s, but the incidence of melanoma has continued to rise considerably in spite of the popularity of sunscreens.

Other potential adverse effects of sunscreen use with regard to melanoma, aside from prolonged exposure to UV radiation, include: (1) interference with the accommodation by the skin to UV light; and (2) interference with the cutaneous synthesis of vitamin D_3.

The research team added that UV-B is the primary signal for an accommodation of skin to sunlight. With the reduced transmission of UV-B, there is less accommodating occurring in those who use sunscreens regularly. Thus, there will be less thickening of the stratum corneum (the outer layer of the epidermis) and less release of melanin-containing granules into the epidermis (tanning), which reduces the transparency to UV-A and UV-B.

Regarding vitamin D_3, skin exposure to UV-B is the principal source of cholecalciferol (vitamin D_3) in most human populations. Sunscreen use has been associated with significant decreases in the synthesis of cholecalciferol (25-hydroxyvitamin D), Garland said.

Obviously, there is much to be learned about sunscreens, how well they protect from the sun's harmful rays, and how they impact on vitamin D synthesis.

24.

Thalassemia

Thalassemia (Mediterranean anemia) is a group of inherited disorders in which there is a defect in the production of hemoglobin, the oxygen-carrying substance that synthesizes in the bone marrow for incorporation into red blood cells, explained the *American Medical Association Home Medical Encyclopedia*. Many of the red blood cells are fragile and quickly break up, leading to hemolytic anemia. This condition is prevalent in people originating from the Mediterranean region, the Middle East, and Southeast Asia.[1]

"The hemoglobin of healthy people contains two pairs of globins or protein chains known as alpha chains and beta chains," the publication said. "In thalassemia, synthesis of either of the chains is reduced, causing an imbalance between alpha and beta chains in much of the hemoglobin that is produced."

Abnormal hemoglobin production in this disorder is caused by inheritance of a defective gene; usually the production of beta chains is disturbed, leading to beta-thalassemia. When people inherit one defective gene for the disease, they are said to have beta-thalassemia minor, or thalassemia trait, which is never severe.

When two defective genes are inherited—one from each parent—the result is much more severe and this is referred to as beta-thalassemia major, or Cooley's anemia. When two people with the minor trait have offspring, each child has a one in four chance of suffering from beta-thalassemia major, the publication added. Cooley's anemia was named after Thomas E. Cooley (1871–1945), an American pediatrician.

Alpha-thalassemia is less common than the beta type. When there is a severely reduced production of alpha chains, the lack of normal hemoglobin is incompatible with life and an affected infant usually dies within a few hours of birth.

Symptoms of beta-thalassemia major involve hemolytic anemia, which include fatigue and shortness of breath, with jaundice and spleen enlargement because of the rapid breakup of red blood cells. These symptoms are usually detected three to six months after birth. If untreated, the bone marrow expands considerably—to compensate for the reduced life span of the red blood cells. This causes bones to grow abnormally, leading to an enlarged skull in untreated patients. Normal body growth is inhibited, and without treatment, death occurs in early childhood. With alpha-thalassemia, anemia is generally less severe, the publication said.

As reported in *Acta Pediatrica,* researchers evaluated two groups of patients with beta-thalassemia, ranging in age from five to ten (fifteen patients) and eleven to twenty-three (twenty-two patients). They found a disturbance in circulating blood levels of 25-hydroxyvitamin D. This disturbance was aggravated as the patients aged.[2]

The research team also found that circulating 24,25(OH)D levels were significantly low in both groups. Abnormally low 25-hydroxyvitamin D—less than 7 ng/dl—was seen in some adolescent patients during winter months, when the vitamin is scarce. The researchers suggested that vitamin D supplementation may be necessary in beta-thalassemia patients, especially during the winter.

25.

Weight Loss

In an article in the *American Journal of Clinical Nutrition,* a research team evaluated nineteen healthy white volunteers of normal body weight and compared them with nineteen obese people with body mass indexes over 30. Those with a body mass index (BMI) over 35 are said to be twenty times as likely to develop diabetes as are those with a BMI between 18.5 and 24.9.[1]

It was reported that the obese volunteers had significantly lower 25-hydroxyvitamin D concentrations and higher parathyroid hormone concentrations than did the controls. Blood levels of vitamin D_3 twenty-four hours after whole-body irradiation revealed a 57 percent lower incremental increase in vitamin D_3 in obese people, compared with nonobese individuals.

It was also reported that the BMI was inversely correlated with blood levels of vitamin D_3 after irradiation and with peak serum vitamin D_2 concentrations, following vitamin D_2 intake at a single dose of 50,000 IU (1.25 mg) given orally. Vitamin D insufficiency related to obesity is probably due to a reduction in the bioavailability of vitamin D_3 from cutaneous and dietary sources because of its storage in body fat compartments, the researchers said.

It has been shown that overweight people with low calcium and dairy consumption were at much greater risk of developing the metabolic syndrome over a ten-year follow-up than were overweight people with high calcium and dairy consumption, reported Geneviève C. Major of Laval University in Ste-Foy, Canada, and colleagues at other locations. This finding suggests that adequate calcium intake could exert a significant effect on the predisposition to a healthier metabolic profile, similar to that of a macronutrient-balanced diet and regular physical activity.[2, 3, 4, 5]

Formerly called Syndrome X, metabolic syndrome is a collection of five conditions that put people at risk for type 2 diabetes and cardiovascular disease.

Those with three or more of these conditions are susceptible to diabetes and cardiovascular disease: (1) a waistline measuring greater than thirty-nine inches (99cm) in men and women (obesity); (2) high blood pressure; (3) high fasting glucose levels; (4) low HDL-cholesterol levels—the beneficial kind; and (5) high triglyceride levels.

The objective of the Major et al study was to determine the effects of daily calcium intake and of supplementation with calcium and vitamin D during a weight loss intervention on blood pressure, plasma lipid, and lipoprotein concentrations and glucose and insulin concentrations in low calcium consumers.

In the Major et al study, sixty-three overweight or obese women with a daily calcium intake of around 800 mg/day were randomly assigned in a double-blind manner to one of two groups. One group was given two tablets a day of a calcium–vitamin D supplement—600 mg of elemental calcium and 200 IU of vitamin D. The other group received a placebo or look-alike pill. Both groups observed a 700 kcal/day energy restriction. The women then completed a fifteen-week weight loss intervention trial.

The Major and colleagues research team reported that initial daily calcium intake was significantly correlated with plasma HDL cholesterol and with a two-hour postload glycemia during an oral glucose tolerance test, independent of fat mass and waist circumference.

Following a fifteen-week intervention, significantly greater decreases in total LDL, LDL-HDL, and LDL cholesterol were noted in the calcium–vitamin D group as opposed to the placebo group. The differences in total HDL and LDL-HDL were independent of changes in fat mass and in waist circumference. A tendency for more beneficial changes in HDL-cholesterol, triglycerides, and total cholesterol was also observed in the calcium–vitamin D group.

"Our results show that consumption of a calcium–vitamin D supplement enhances the beneficial effect of body weight loss on the lipid and lipoprotein profile in overweight or obese women with usual low calcium intake," the researchers said. "Future research should be oriented toward a better understanding of the effect of a usual insufficient calcium intake on the expected outcome of a supplementation with calcium and more specifically with respect to its effect on glucose and insulin and blood pressure variables."

Major and colleagues added that between weeks zero and fourteen, there was a decrease in body weight, body mass index, waist circumference, and fat mass. In addition, plasma triglyceride concentrations decreased in the calcium–vitamin D group, but increased in the placebo group.

THE FATTEST STATES

Obesity contributes to diabetes, heart disease, and other life-threatening illnesses. Here are the obesity rankings, by state, from 2004–2006.

1. Mississippi	18. Nebraska	35. Wyoming
2. West Virginia	19. North Dakota	36. California
3. Alabama	20. Iowa	37. Nevada
4. Louisiana	21. South Dakota	38. New Hampshire
5. South Carolina	22. Wisconsin	39. New York
6. Tennessee	23. Pennsylvania	40. District of Columbia
7. Kentucky	24. Virginia	41. New Jersey
8. Arkansas	25. Illinois	42. New Mexico
9. Indiana	26. Maryland	43. Arizona
10. Michigan	27. Kansas	44. Utah
11. Oklahoma	28. Minnesota	45. Montana
12. Missouri	29. Delaware	46. Rhode Island
13. Texas	30. Oregon	47. Connecticut
14. Georgia	31. Idaho	48. Hawaii
15. Ohio	32. Washington	49. Vermont
16. Alaska	33. Maine	50. Massachusetts
17. North Carolina	34. Florida	51. Colorado

Source: "Living Large," *AAHP Bulletin* 48, no. 10 (November 2007): 29.

26.

How Safe Is Vitamin D?

Various arguments favoring higher intakes of calcium and other nutrients have been based on evidence about the diets of prehistoric humans; the circulating levels of 25-hydroxyvitamin D (25(OH)D) in the blood of our ancestors were surely higher than what is now regarded as normal, explained Reinhold Vieth, PhD, of the University of Toronto.[1]

As an example, the full body surface of our ancestors was exposed to the sun almost daily, in contrast to modern humans who cover all but about 5 percent of our body surface, and it is rare for us to spend time in unshielded sunlight. For adults, the 200 IU/day vitamin D recommended dietary allowance may prevent osteomalacia in the absence of sunlight, but more is needed to help prevent osteoporosis and secondary hyperparathyroidism, Vieth continued.

"Total body sun exposure easily provides the equivalent of 10,000 IU/day of vitamin D (250 mcg), suggesting that this is a physiologic limit," he added. "To insure that serum 25(OH)D concentrations exceed 100 nmol/l, a total vitamin D supply of 4,000 IU/day (100 mcg) is required."

He goes on to say that, except in those with conditions causing hypersensitivity, there is no evidence of adverse effects with serum 25(OH)D concentrations less than 140 nmol/l, which require a total vitamin D supply of 10,000 IU/day to attain.

"Published cases of vitamin D toxicity with hypercalcemia, for which the 25(OH)D concentration and vitamin D dose are known, all involve intake of over 1,000 mcg (40,000 IU/day)," Vieth said. "Because vitamin D is potentially toxic, intake of 1,000 IU/day (over 25 mcg) has been avoided, even though the weight of evidence shows that the currently accepted observed adverse effect limit of 50 mcg (2,000 IU/day) is too low by at least five fold."

The current adult daily reference intake (DRI) for vitamin D approximates half the amount in the teaspoon of cod-liver oil, which was used as a nineteenth-century folk remedy, Vieth continued. New drugs are passed through dose-finding studies before their efficacy is evaluated in clinical trials, but this principle is not strictly applicable to nutrient recommendations, because the bulk of what humans consume is from unfortified foods and this consumption is what recommended intakes tend to match.

"In contrast," Vieth said, "vitamin D is a special case, in that the bulk of our dietary vitamin D intake is determined by legislation. I contend that this practice amounts to the dosing of populations with a drug—vitamin D—that is not present in the foods humans normally consume."

If vitamin D is similar to a drug, he continued, then dose-finding studies are needed to use it properly, especially if nonclassical benefits are potentially relevant. If vitamin D is contrasted with other nutrients, and vitamin D supplementation is intended to make up for what some people may not be getting from its natural source—the sun—then the current adult DRI of 200 IU/day is woefully inadequate, he said.

New clinical research results over the past ten years indicate that the approximate intakes of vitamin D may provide greater health benefits than previously thought, benefits that include not only improved bone health, but also other effects as well, reported John N. Hathcock, PhD, of the Council for Responsible Nutrition in Washington, D.C., and his colleagues, Andrew Shao, Reinhold Vieth, and Robert Heaney. However, the amounts of vitamin D needed to produce beneficial effects are greater than previously thought. Unfortunately, the adequate intakes of 200–600 IU/day of vitamin D for adults nineteen years of age and older, as expressed by the Food and Nutrition Board, is based on older evidence, they reported in the *American Journal of Clinical Nutrition* in 2007.[2]

"Safety is always an important consideration when formulating recommendations for nutrient intake," the researchers said. "The just-named Board evaluated the potential for high intakes of the vitamin to produce adverse effects and set a safe limit of 2,000 IU/day (50 mcg). Using similar methodology, the European Commission Scientific Committee on Food (SCF) also identified the safe upper limit for vitamin D. However, though a less quantitative application of the same method, the United Kingdom Expert Group on Vitamins and Minerals (EVM) set a vitamin D_3 upper limit of 25 mcg (1,000 IU/day)."

The researchers provide an extensive review of all the relevant human and animal studies concerning the safety of vitamin D. The criterion for study inclusion was the use of a vitamin D dose substantially above the current 1,800

IU/day, followed by study design, duration, and sample size. Relevant outcomes include statistically significant changes in serum 25(OH)D and increases in urinary calcium, serum calcium, or both.

"Unfortified foods, fortified foods, and most dietary supplements combined do not contribute to a total exposure anywhere near the recommended vitamin D upper limit of 250 mcg/day," the researchers added. "There is little prospect of exposure of the healthy general population to toxic levels of vitamin D with current or likely levels in fortified foods and dietary supplements. Therefore, total exposure to vitamin D, including an autogenous production under UV light stimulation, is very unlikely to exceed this proposed upper limit value."

They added that combining this proposed upper limit with total erythemic sunlight exposure and typical dietary and supplemental sources all at once would still result in a serum 25(OH)D concentration of around 500 nmol/l, which is well below the estimated concentration associated with hypercalcemia, which is over 600 nmol/l.

Indeed, they continued, there is a lot of room for increased vitamin D intakes without risk of overdose. Much larger amounts, such as 2,500 mcg, have shown no toxicity if restricted to one occasion per four months or daily for a single period of four/day.

In a previous publication, *Vitamin and Mineral Safety*, Hathcock said that, in most adults, daily intake in excess of 50,000 IU (1.25 mg) of vitamin D is needed to produce toxicity (Miller and Hayes, 1982—see note 4 in this chapter). However, lower amounts may cause problems for those with sarcoidosis (nodules in lymph nodes, lungs, etc.), myobacterial infections like TB, or idiopathic hypercalcemia, and toxicity can occur at levels of vitamin D intake only somewhat above normal—over 25 mcg/day (1,000 IU).[3,4]

"A causal relationship between excess vitamin D intake and idiopathic hypercalcemia is unlikely, although people with idiopathic calcemia may be subject to adverse effects of vitamin D at lower intakes than those who are normal," Hathcock said.

He added that, in children of unreported body weight—between 10 and 30 kg—the amount of dietary vitamin D that has led to adverse effects may be as low as 2,000–4,000 IU/day. In full-term infants, adverse effects have been reported with intakes as low as 1,800 IU/day; however, no adverse effects occurred in a six-month study of infants given 1,600 IU/day.

As noted throughout this book, scientists are still unraveling the mysteries of vitamin D. From all the available evidence, many of us are not getting the required amounts of the vitamin from the sun, diet, and supplements, which leave us vulnerable to a host of life-threatening illnesses.

Glossary

Adenocarcinoma: A glandular cancer.

Albumin: The most abundant protein in the body. It is made in the liver from amino acids.

Albuterol: A bronchodilator.

Alveolar: Part of the jaw where the teeth arise.

Amenorrhea: Cessation of the menses.

Amyotrophic lateral sclerosis (ALS): One of a group of diseases in which the nerves that control muscular activity degenerate within the brain and spinal cord. Also known as Lou Gehrig's disease.

Angiogenesis: Development of new blood vessels.

Ankylosing spondylitis: An inflammatory disease affecting joints between the vertebra of the spine and sacroiliac joints.

Anorexia nervosa: An eating disorder in which the sufferer fears becoming obese and consequently starves herself (most common in females).

Anus: Posterior opening of the alimentary canal.

Articular: Relating to a joint.

Asthma: An illness characterized by recurrent attacks of breathlessness, accompanied by wheezing.

Atrophy: Wasting of tissues, organs, etc.

Betamethasone: A glucocorticoid with anti-inflammatory effects.

Biopsy: The removal of cells for examination under a microscope.

Bone mineral density (BMD): A risk factor for fractures. Usually expressed as the amount of mineralized tissue in the area scanned (g/cm^2); with some technologies, expressed as amount per volume of bone (g/cm^3). Hip BMD, considered the best predictor of hip fracture, appears to predict other types of fractures as well as measurements made at other skeletal sites. Spine BMD may be preferable to assess changes early in menopause and after bilateral ovariectomy (removal of one or both ovaries).

Calcidiol: 25-hydroxycholecalciferol.

Calcifediol: *See* Calcidiol.

Calciferol: *See* Ergocalciferol (vitamin D_2).

Calcitonin: A polypeptide hormone that inhibits the resorptive activity of osteoclasts. Because of its analgesic effect, it is frequently used for patients with acute, symptomatic vertebral fractures. Studies indicate that calcitonin may decrease vertebral fractures by about two-thirds.

Calcitriol: A synthetic form of 1,25-dihydroxyvitamin D_3, a hormone that aids calcium absorption and mineralization of the skeleton. Its effectiveness as a treatment for osteoporosis is still being evaluated.

Calcium: A mineral that plays an essential role in the development and maintenance of a healthy skeleton. If a person's calcium intake is inadequate, calcium is mobilized (leached) from the skeleton to maintain a normal blood calcium level. In addition to being a substrate for bone mineralization, calcium has an inhibitory effect on bone remodeling through suppression of circulating parathyroid hormone.

Cancellous bone: The spongy or trabecular tissue in the middle of bone (e.g., vertebrae) and at the end of long bones.

Celiac disease: Also known as gluten intolerance. An illness in which the small intestine is damaged by gluten, a protein found in wheat, rye, oats, and barley. Some sufferers can tolerate oats, millet, etc.

Chondroblast: A dividing cell of growing cartilage tissue.

Chondrocyte: A cartilage cell.

Chondroitin sulfate: A mucopolysaccharide found in connective tissue.

Cirrhosis: A liver disease caused by chronic damage to the cells; usually associated with alcoholism.

Colonoscopy: An examination of the inside of the colon, the major part of the large intestine.

Cortical bone: The dense outer layer of bone.

C-reactive protein: A protein found in blood serum.

Creatinine: A compound found in blood, muscle, and urine.

Crohn's disease: An inflammatory disease that affects the gastrointestinal tract from the mouth to the anus.

Cystic fibrosis (CF): An inherited disease; sufferers have a tendency to contract chronic lung infections and have an inability to absorb fats and other nutrients in food.

Cytokines: Substances secreted by cells of the immune system.

Cytomegalo virus: A group of viruses affecting the salivary glands.

7-dehydrocholesterol: Provitamin D_3.

Dermis: The skin layer below the epidermis.

Diatom: Unicellular algae.

1a,25-dihydroxycholecalciferol: An active form of vitamin D.

1,25-dihydroxyergocalciferol: An active metabolite of vitamin D_2.

1a,25-dihydroxyvitamin D (1,25(OH2)D: Vitamin D.

1,25-dihydroxyvitamin D_3 (1,25(OH)$_2$D$_3$): Vitamin D.

Dithranol (anthralin): Compounds obtained from coal tar.

Dual energy x-ray absorptionmetry (DXA or DEXA): A diagnostic test used to assess bone density in the spine, hip, or wrist, using radiation exposure about one-tenth that of a standard chest x-ray.

Eczema: An inflammation of the skin, often causing scaling or blisters.

Edema: An accumulation of fluid; swelling.

Enterovirus: A group of viruses that inhabit the alimentary canal.

Epidermis: The protective epithelial outer portion of the skin.

Ergocalciferol: Vitamin D_2.

25-ergocalciferol: Vitamin D_2.

Ergosterol: A crystalline sterol alcohol in yeast, molds, and ergot (fungi), which is converted by UV radiation into vitamin D_2.

Estrogen: One of a group of steroid hormones that control female sexual development. Estrogen directly affects bone mass through estrogen receptors in bone, reducing bone turnover and bone loss. It indirectly increases intestinal calcium absorption and kidney calcium conservation and, therefore, calcium balance. *See* Hormone replacement therapy.

Family history: A risk factor for osteoporotic fractures, defined as a maternal and/or paternal history of hip, wrist, or spine fracture when the parent was fifty or older.

Fistula: An abnormal passage leading from one hollow surface to another.

Fracture: Breakage of a bone, either complete or incomplete. Most studies of osteoporosis focus on hip, vertebra, and/or wrist fractures.

Gingivitis: Gum disease.

Glucocorticoids: Steroids prescribed for their anti-inflammatory effect.

Hemoglobin A1C: This is formed when glucose becomes attached to hemoglobin molecules. The quantity formed serves as an indicator of average blood sugar levels for the eight- to twelve-week period prior to the test.

Homeostasis: Balance.

Hormone: A chemical substance formed in an organ or part of the body and carried by the blood to another organ.

Hormone replacement therapy (HRT): A general term for all types of estrogen replacement therapy when given with progestin, cyclically or continuously. HRT is generally prescribed for women after natural menopause or bilateral oviarectomy. Studies indicate that five years of HRT may decrease vertebral fractures by 50 to 80 percent and nonvertebral fractures by about 25 percent. Ten or more years of use might be expected to decrease the rate of all fractures by 50 to 75 percent. Since there are ominous side effects associated with HRT (weight gain, blood clots, breast cancer, etc.), check with your doctor about using it.

Hydrolysis: The chemical process by which a substance unites with water and then divides into smaller molecules.

25-hydroxycholecalciferol: Calcidiol.

Hydroxylation: Putting a hydroxyl group in a substance where one did not exist before.

Hyperalimentation: Giving nutrients via intravenous feeding.

Hypercalcemia: High amounts of calcium in the blood.

Hypercalciuria: Excretion of large amounts of calcium in the urine.

Hypercholesterolemia: Abnormally large amounts of cholesterol in cells and blood.

Hyperglycemia: High amounts of glucose in the blood.

Hyperinsulinemia: Increased amounts of insulin in the blood.

Hyperparathyroidism: Overactivity of the parathyroid glands.

Hyperphosphatemia: High amounts of phosphates in the blood.

Hyperthyroidism: Abnormal secretion of the thyroid hormone.

Hypertrophy: Exaggerated growth of an organ.

Hypoglycemia: Low amount of glucose circulating in the blood. Also known as low blood sugar.

Hypogonadism: Inadequate gonadal function.

Hypothermia: Body temperature below 98.6°F (37°C).

Ileum: Lower portion of the small intestine.

Inguinal: Relating to the groin.

Insulin: A hormone released by the beta cells of the pancreas.

Insulin resistance: A condition in which the body does not respond to insulin produced by the pancreas, leading to type 2 diabetes.

Islets of Langerhans: Special groups of cells in the pancreas that make and secrete hormones that help the body break down and use food. They include beta cells, alpha cells, delta cells, PP cells, and D1 cells.

IU: International Unit.

Keratin: Fibrous protein such as hair, nails, etc.

Ketoacidosis: A severe condition, usually in type 1 diabetes, caused by insufficient insulin.

Kyphoplasty: Minimally invasive surgical treatment for pain management following vertebral body compression fractures; associated with osteoporosis.

Kyphosis: Abnormal forward curvature of the spine.

Lactose-intolerant: Lacking the enzyme lactase to digest the lactose in milk.

Lou Gehrig's disease: *See* Amyotrophic lateral sclerosis.

Low bone mass (osteopenia): The designation for bone density between 1.0 and 2.5 standard deviations below the mean for young, normal adults (T-score between –1 and 2.5).

Lumen: The space in the interior of an artery, intestine, etc.

Lymphocytes: White blood cells.

Lymphokines: Hormonelike peptides, activated by lymphocytes, which mediate immune responses.

Macrophages: Phagocytic tissue cells that attack and ingest germs and other foreign bodies.

Mast cells: Connective tissues.

Mcg: Microgram, one-millionth of a gram.

Melanoma: The most serious type of three skin cancers (the other two being basal cell carcinoma and squamous cell carcinoma).

Mercaptopurine: An antimetabolite that interferes with purine synthesis. Also known as 6-MP.

Metabolic syndrome: Formerly called *Syndrome X.* A cluster of independent risk factors: impaired glucose regulation, central obesity, high levels of cholesterol in the blood, high levels of triglycerides in the blood, and high blood pressure. Anyone with three of the five risk factors may be a candidate for diabetes or cardiovascular disease.

Metalloprotein: Hemoglobin.

Mg: Milligram; one-thousandth of a gram.

Modeling: The term for processes that occur during growth and increase in bone mass, such as linear growth, cortical apposition, and cancellous modification.

Mucolytic: Capable of dissolving or digesting mucus.

Multiple sclerosis (MS): A disease of the central nervous system in which scattered patches of myelin—the protective covering of nerve fibers—in the brain and spinal cord are destroyed.

Myopathy: A disease of the muscles.

Neuropathy: A disorder affecting the nervous system.

Nephropathy: Kidney disease.

Neutrophil: A mature white blood cell.

Ng: Nanogram; one-billionth of a gram.

Nm: Nanometer, one-billionth of a meter.

Non-Hodgkin's lymphoma: A malignant form of lymphoma, such as Birkitt's lymphoma.

Normal bone mass: The designation for bone density within one standard deviation of the mean for young, normal, adult women (T-score above −1).

N-telepeptide: A marker for bone resorption.

Nulliparous: Referring to a woman who has never given birth.

Osteoarthritis: Erosion of articular cartilage due to trauma or other conditions, which become soft, frayed, and thinned.

Osteoblast: A bone-forming cell derived from a fibroblast.

Osteocalcin: A protein found in bone and dentin.

Osteocetasis: Bowing of bones, especially in the legs.

Osteochondritis: Inflammation of a bone or cartilage.

Osteoclast: A large, multinucleated cell.

Osteogenesis: The formation of bone.

Osteohypertrophy: Overgrowth of bones.

Osteoid: Referring to newly formed organic bone prior to calcification.

Osteomalacia: A disease characterized by a gradual softening and bending of bones, often due to a vitamin D deficiency. *See* Rickets.

Osteopenia: A condition involving reduced bone mass due to inadequate osteoid synthesis.

Osteophyte: A bony outgrowth.

Osteoporosis: A chronic, progressive disease characterized by low bone mass and microarchitectural deterioration of bone tissue, leading to bone fragility and a consequent increase in fracture risk; bone density more than 2.5 standard deviations below the young, normal mean (T-score below −2.5).

Parathyroid glands: Four glands embedded in the thyroid gland. The hormones secreted by these glands control calcium and phosphorus levels.

Parathyroid hormone (PTH): A hormone, secreted by the parathyroid glands, which promotes the passage in the urine of phosphates, a decrease of phosphates in blood plasma, and an increase in blood calcium.

Pancreas: A gland extending from the duodenum to the spleen. It secretes juices to aid digestion.

Pancreatitis: Inflammation of the pancreas.

Patella: Kneecap.

Pathognomic: Denoting a disease.

Peak bone mass: The maximum bone mass accumulated during youth.

Periodontal disease: A disease of the gums, caused by dental plaque and characterized by gingival inflammation.

Periosteum: Connective tissue around a bone.

Peripheral fractures: Nonvertebral fractures; that is, those of the hip, wrist, forearm, leg, ankle, feet, rib, sternum, and other sites.

Pg: Picogram; one-trillionth of a gram.

Phagocytes: Cells that ingest bacteria and other foreign substances.

Pmol: Picomole; one-trillionth of a mole.

Polymorphisms: Instances of something occurring in more than one form.

Postmenopausal: Referring to the period following menopause.

Previous fracture: A risk factor for fractures, defined as a history of previous fractures after age forty.

Proteoglycans: Found in the extracellular matrix of connective tissue.

Psoriasis: A skin disease characterized by thickened patches of inflamed, red skin.

Quantitative computed tomography (QCT): A diagnostic test used to assess bone density. It reflects three-dimensional bone mineral density. Usually used to assess the lumbar spine, but it has been adapted for other skeletal sites.

Rachitic: Relating to rickets.

Radiographic absorptiometry (RA): A diagnostic test used to assess bone density at a peripheral site, usually the hand. Such techniques are referred to as an aluminum equivalence, photodensitometry, and radiographic densitometry.

Remodeling: The ongoing dual processes of bone formation and bone resorption after cessation of growth.

Resorption: The loss of a substance, such as bone, through physiological or pathological means.

Retinol: Vitamin A.

Rickets: An illness caused by a vitamin D deficiency; characterized by overproduction and deficient calcification of osteoid tissue.

Sarcopenia: The involuntary decline in lean body mass that occurs with age, primarily due to loss of skeletal muscle.

Scleroderma: Thickening of the skin and other tissues due to new collagen formation. It is marked by the disposition of fibrous connective tissue in the skin and often in internal organs as well.

Secondary osteoporosis: Osteoporosis that is drug-induced or is caused by disorders such as hyperthyroidism, kidney disease, or chronic obstructive pulmonary disease.

Severe or "established" osteoporosis: Osteoporosis characterized by bone density that is more than 2.5 standard deviations below the young normal range (T-score below −2.5), accompanied by the occurrence of at least one fragility-related fracture.

Sigmoidoscopy: Examination of the sigmoid colon and rectum with a sigmoidoscope.

Single x-ray absorptiometry (SXA): A diagnostic test used to assess bone density. Limited to peripheral sites, it cannot measure bone density in the hip or spine, nor can it discriminate between cortical and cancellous bone.

Stratum corneum: The outer, horny layer of the epidermis.

Stratum lucidum: Clear layer of the epidermis.

Stroma: Connective tissue of a gland, organ, etc.

Synovia: A transparent lubricating fluid in a joint cavity.

Tetany: A neurological syndrome causing muscle twitches, cramps, etc.

Thalassemia: A disease occurring in the Mediterranean region and characterized by enlargement of the spleen, anemia, and changes in the bones, with pigmentation of the skin. Also called Cooley's anemia.

Thyrotoxicosis: Production of too much thyroid hormone.

Trabecula: A spongy substance in bone.

Trochanter: Rough prominence at the upper part of the femur.

T-score: In describing bone mineral density, the number of standard deviations above or below the mean for young, normal adults.

Type 1 diabetes: Formerly called juvenile diabetes or insulin-dependent diabetes.

Type 2 diabetes: Formerly known as adult-onset diabetes or non–insulin-dependent diabetes.

Ulcerative colitis: Chronic inflammation of the lining of the colon and rectum.

Ulna: The larger and inner of the two bones of the forearm; on the side of the small finger.

Ultrasound densitometry: A diagnostic test used to assess bone density at the calcaneus or patella. Ultrasound measurements correlated only modestly with other assessments of bone density in the same patients. However, some prospective studies indicate that ultrasound may predict fractures as well as other measures of bone density.

Vertebra: One of the segments of the spinal column. There are usually thirty-three vertebrae: seven cervical, twelve thoracic, five lumbar, five sacral—fused into one bone (the sacrum), and four coccygeal—fused into one bone (the coccyx).

Vertebroplasty: A minimally invasive procedure designed to relieve the pain of vertebral compression fractures associated with osteoporosis.

Vitamin D$_2$: *See* Ergocalciferol.

Vitamin D$_3$: *See* Cholecalciferol.

Z-score: In describing bone mineral density, the number of standard deviations above or below the mean for persons of the same age.

Notes

Chapter 1

1. Michael F. Holick, MD, "Vitamin D: Importance in the Prevention of Cancers, Type 1 Diabetes, Heart Disease, and Osteoporosis," *American Journal of Clinical Nutrition* 79 (2004): 362–371.

2. Robert P. Heaney, MD, "Long-Latency Definition: Insights from Calcium and Vitamin D," *American Journal of Clinical Nutrition* 78 (2003): 912–919.

3. Audrey H. Ensminger et al., *Foods & Nutrition Encyclopedia* (Clovis, CA: Pegus Press, 1983), pp. 2256ff.

4. Food and Nutrition Board, National Research Council, *Recommended Dietary Allowances,* 10th ed. (Washington, D.C.: National Academy Press, 1989), pp. 92ff.

5. Heaney, "Long-Latency Definition."

6. Kirk Hamilton, "Vitamin D, Safety and Chronic Disease," *Clinical Pearls* (Sacramento: IT Services, 1999), pp. 110–111. *Also,* Reinhold Vieth, PhD, "Vitamin D Supplementation, 25-Hydroxyvitamin D Concentrations, and Safety," *American Journal of Clinical Nutrition* 69 (1999): 842–856.

7. Claudia Dreyfus, "Shining a Light on the Health Benefits of Vitamin D," *New York Times* (January 28, 2003), p. F5.

8. Bill Marsh, "A Need That Doesn't Change with the Seasons," *New York Times* (January 28, 2003): F5.

9. Robert P. Heaney, MD, "Lessons for Nutritional Science from Vitamin D," *American Journal of Clinical Nutrition* 69 (1999): 825–826.

10. A. M. Parfitt, "Osteomalacia and Related Disorders," in Avioli et al., *Metabolic Bone Disease and Clinically Related Disorders,* 2nd ed. (Philadelphia: W.B. Saunders, 1990), pp. 329–396.

11. Vieth, "Vitamin D Supplementation, 25-Hydroxyvitamin D Concentrations, and Safety."

12. Heike A. Bischoff-Ferrari et al., "Estimation of Optimal Serum Concentrations of 25-Hydroxyvitamin D for Multiple Health Outcomes," *American Journal of Clinical Nutrition* 84 (2006): 18–28.

13. Robert P. Heaney, MD, "Calcium Absorption Varies within the Reference Range for Serum 25-Hydroxyvitamin D," *Journal of the American College of Nutrition* 22 (2003): 142–146.

14. A. Devine et al., "Effects of Vitamin D Metabolism on Intestinal Calcium Absorption and Bone Turnover in Elderly Women," *American Journal of Clinical Nutrition* 75 (2002): 283–288.

15. Melissa K. Thomas, MD, PhD, et al., "Hypovitaminosis D in Medical Inpatients," *New England Journal of Medicine* 338, no. 12 (1998): 777–783.

16. Hennie C. J. P. Janssen et al., "Vitamin D Deficiency, Muscle Function, and Falls in Elderly People," *American Journal of Clinical Nutrition* 75 (2002): 611–615.

17. G. D. Schott and M. R. Willis, "Muscle Weakness in Osteomalacia," *Lancet* 1 (1976): 626–629.

18. F. M. Gloth III et al., "Vitamin D Deficiency in Housebound Elderly Persons," *JAMA* 274 (1995): 1683–1686.

19. Mark J. Bolland et al., "The Effects of Seasonal Variation of 25-Hydroxyvitamin D and Fat Mass on a Diagnosis of Vitamin D Deficiency," *American Journal of Clinical Nutrition* 86 (2007): 959–964.

20. P. Autier and S. Gandini, "Vitamin D Supplementation and Total Mortality: A Meta-Analysis of Randomized Controlled Trials," *Archives of Internal Medicine* 167 (2007): 1730–1737.

21. "Supplements Could Save U.S. $24 Billion," *Whole Foods Magazine* (July 2007): 9.

22. Paul F. Jacques, PhD, et al., "Plasma 25-Hydroxyvitamin D and its Determinants in an Elderly Population Sample," *American Journal of Clinical Nutrition* 66 (1997): 929–936.

23. Ruth Adams, *The Complete Home Guide to All the Vitamins* (New York: Larchmont Books, 1979), p. 314.

24. M. Karkkainen et al., "Low Serum Vitamin D Concentrations and Secondary Hyperparathyroidism in Middle Aged, Caucasian Strict Vegetarians," *Challenges of Modern Medicine* 7 (1995): 342–344.

25. Edward B. Blau, "Congenital Cataracts and Maternal Vitamin D Deficiency," *Lancet* 347, no. 2 (March 2, 1996): 626.

26. William A. Bauman, MD, et al., "Vitamin D Deficiency in Veterans with Chronic Spinal Cord Injury," *Metabolism* 44, no. 12 (December 1995): 1612–1616.

27. Richard C. Henderson, MD, PhD "Vitamin D Levels in Non-Institutionalized Children with Cerebral Palsy," *Journal of Child Neurology* 12 (1997): 443–447.

28. Joan Stephenson, PhD "Vitamin D and Pregnancy," *JAMA* 295, no. 7 (2006): 748.

29. Mary E. Mohs, PhD, RD, "Nutritional Effects of Marijuana, Heroin, Cocaine, and Nicotine," *Journal of the American Dietetic Association* 90 (1990): 1261–1267.

30. R. J. Wilkinson et al., "Influence of Vitamin D Deficiency and Vitamin D Receptor Polymorphisms on Tuberculosis among Gujarati Asians in West London: A Case Control Study," *Lancet* 355 (February 19, 2000): 618–621.

31. A. T. G. Landsdowne and S. C. Provost, "Vitamin D Enhances Mood in Healthy Subjects during Winter," *Psychopharmacology* 135 (1998): 319–323.

32. J. McGrath, "Hypothesis: Is Low Prenatal Vitamin D a Risk Modifying Factor for Schizophrenia?" *Schizophrenic Research* 40 (1999): 173–177.

33. Shanna Nesby-O'Dell et al., "Hypovitaminosis D Prevalence and Determinants among African American and White Women of Reproductive Age: Third National Health and Nutrition Examination Survey, 1988–1994," *American Journal of Clinical Nutrition* 76 (2002): 187–192.

34. H. M. Perry et al., "Aging and Bone Metabolism in African American and Caucasian Women," *Journal of Clinical Endocrinology and Metabolism* 81 (1996): 1108–1117.

35. J. B. Dibble et al., "A Survey of Vitamin D Deficiency in Gastrointestinal and Liver Disorders," *Quarterly Journal of Medicine* 209 (Winter 1984): 119–134.

Chapter 2

1. Karen Collins, MS, RD, "The Latest Lessons on Calcium and Vitamin D," *American Institute for Cancer Research,* Washington, D.C., June 5, 2006.

2. Yannis Manios et al., "Changes in Biochemical Indexes of Bone Metabolism and Bone Mineral Density, after a 12 Month Dietary Intervention Program: The Postmenopausal Health Study," *American Journal of Clinical Nutrition* 86 (2007): 781–789.

3. Laufey Steingrimsdottir, PhD, et al., "Relationship between Serum Parathyroid Hormone Levels, Vitamin D Deficiency, and Calcium Intake," *JAMA* 294, no. 18 (2005): 2336–2441.

4. Robert D. Utiger, MD, "The Need for More Vitamin D," *New England Journal of Medicine* 338, no. 12 (1998): 828–829.

5. Mariana Cifuentes et al., "Weight Loss and Calcium Intake Influence Calcium Absorption in Overweight Postmenopausal Women," *American Journal of Clinical Nutrition* 80 (2004): 123–130.

6. Horace M. Perry III et al., "A Preliminary Report of Vitamin D and Calcium Metabolism in Older African Americans," *Journal of the American Geriatrics Society* 41 (1993): 612–616.

7. I. R. Reid, "The Roles of Calcium and Vitamin D in the Prevention of Osteoporosis," *Endocrinology and Metabolism Clinics of North America* 27, no. 2 (June 1998): 389–398.

8. Bess Dawson-Hughes, MD, "Calcium and Vitamin D Nutritional Needs of Elderly Women," *Journal of Nutrition* 126 (1996): 1165S–1167S.

9. H. Karimi Kinyamu et al., "Dietary Calcium and Vitamin D Intake in Elderly Women: Effect on Serum Parathyroid Hormone and Vitamin D Metabolites," *American Journal of Clinical Nutrition* 67(1998): 342–348.

Chapter 3

1. Bruce W. Hollis and Carol L. Wagner, "Assessment of Dietary Vitamin D Requirements during Pregnancy and Lactation," *American Journal of Clinical Nutrition* 79 (2004): 717–726.

2. L. Cancela et al., "Relationship between the Vitamin D Content of Maternal Milk and the Vitamin D Status of Nursing Women and Breastfed Infants," *Journal of Endocrinology* 110 (1986): 43–50.

3. F. R. Greer and S. Marshall, "Bone Mineral Content, Serum Vitamin Metabolism Concentrations and Ultraviolet-B Light Exposure to Infants Fed Human Milk with and without Vitamin D Supplementations," *Journal of Pediatrics* 114 (1989): 204–212.

4. Reinhold Vieth et al., "Efficiency and Safety of Vitamin D_3 Intake Exceeding the Lowest Observed Adverse Effect Level (LOAEL)," *American Journal of Clinical Nutrition* 73 (2001): 288–292.

5. R. P. Heaney et al., "Human Serum 25-Hydroxycholecalciferol Response to Extended Oral Dosing with Cholecalciferol," *American Journal of Clinical Nutrition* 77 (2003): 204–210.

6. Carlos A. Camargo Jr. et al. "Maternal Intake of Vitamin D during Pregnancy and Risk of Recurrent Wheeze in Children at 3 Years of Age," *American Journal of Clinical Nutrition* 85 (2007): 788–795.

7. Eric Nagourney, "Supplements May Help Prevent Stress Fractures," *New York Times* (February 20, 2007): F6.

8. Hussein F. Saadi et al. "Efficacy of Daily and Monthly High Dose Calciferol in Vitamin D Deficient Nulliaporous and Lactating Women," *American Journal of Clinical Nutrition* 85 (2007): 1565–1571.

9. Puneet Arora and Ramandeep S. Arora, "Vitamin D Supplementation for Non-Western Pregnant Women: The British Experience," *American Journal of Clinical Nutrition* 85 (2007): 1164–1165.

10. I. M. van der Meer et al., "High Prevalence of Vitamin D Deficiency in Pregnant Non-Western Women in The Hague," *American Journal of Clinical Nutrition* 84 (2006): 350–353.

11. M. Ito et al., "Prevention of Preeclampsia with Calcium Supplementation and Vitamin D_3 in Antenatal Protocol," *International Federation of Gynecology and OBS* 47, no. 2 (1994): 115–120.

12. Dwight P. Cruikshank, MD, et al., "Alterations in Vitamin D and Calcium Metabolism with Magnesium Sulfate Treatment of Preeclampsia," *Journal of Obstetrics and Gynecology* 168, no. 4 (April 1993): 1170–1171.

13. Judy McBride, "More Vitamin D May Benefit Black Women," *USDA Food & Nutrition Research Briefs* (October 1998): 3–4.

14. M. Kyriakidou-Himonas et al., "Vitamin D Supplementation in Postmenopausal Black Women," *Journal of Clinical Endocrinology and Metabolism* 84, no. 11 (1999): 3988–3990.

15. Meryl S. LeBoff, MD, "Occult Vitamin D Deficiency in Postmenopausal U.S. Women with Acute Hip Fractures," *JAMA* 281, no. 16 (1999): 1505–1511.

16. K. A. McAuley, MD, et al., "Low Vitamin D Status Is Common among Elderly Dunedin Women," *New Zealand Medical Journal* 110 (1997): 275–277.

17. A. Morabia et al., "Smoking, Dietary Calcium and Vitamin D Deficiency in Women: A Population Based Study," *European Journal of Clinical Nutrition* 54 (2000): 684–689.

18. Chittari V. Harinarayan et al., "High Prevalence of Low Dietary Calcium, High Phyrate Consumption, and Vitamin D Deficiency in Healthy South Indians," *American Journal of Clinical Nutrition* 85 (2007): 1062–1067.

19. Susan Thys-Jacobs, MD, "Vitamin D and Calcium in Menstrual Migraines," *Headache* 34, no. 9 (October 1994): 544–546.

Chapter 4

1. Catherine M. Willis et al., "A Prospective Analysis of Plasma 25-Hydroxyvitamin D Concentrations in White and Black Pre-pubertal Females in the Northeastern United States," *American Journal of Clinical Nutrition* 85 (2007): 124–130.

2. Michael F. Holick, PhD, MD, "Vitamin D: The Underappreciated D-Lightful Hormone that Is Important for Skeletal and Cellular Health," *Current Opinion in Endocrinology and Diabetest* 9 (2002): 87–98.

3. S. A. Zamora et al., "Vitamin D Supplementation during Infancy Is Associated with Higher Bone Mineral Mass in Prepubertal Girls," *Journal of Clinical Endocrinology and Metabolism* 84 (1999): 4541–4544.

4. "Diet of Teenage Girls May Increase Their Risk of Breast Cancer," *Primary Care and Cancer* 14, no. 2 (1994): 8.

5. "Children's Health," *Health Gems* 7, no. 1 (2006): 10.

6. Francis L. Weng et al., "Risk Factors for Low Serum 25-Hydroxyvitamin D Concentrations in Otherwise Healthy Children and Adolescents," *American Journal of Clinical Nutrition* 86 (2007): 150–158.

7. J. G. Haddad, "Vitamin D—Solar Rays, the Milky Way or Both?" *New England Journal of Medicine* 326 (1992): 1213–1215.

8. Michael F. Holick, PhD, MD, "Vitamin D Importance in the Prevention of Cancers, Type 1 Diabetes, Heart Disease, and Osteoporosis," *American Journal of Clinical Nutrition* 79 (2004): 362–371.

9. Marion Taylor Baer et al., "Vitamin D, Calcium, and Bone Status in Children with Developmental Delay in Relation to Anticonvulsant Use and Ambulatory Status," *American Journal of Clinical Nutrition* 65 (1997): 1042–1051.

10. Francis Mimouni, MD, "Sun Protection and Vitamin D Status in Infants," *American Journal of Diseases of Children* 146 (November 1992): 1260.

11. Terhi A. Outila et al., "Vitamin D Status Affects Serum Parathyroid Hormone Concentrations during Winter in Female Adolescents: Associations with Forearm Bone Mineral Density," *American Journal of Clinical Nutrition* 74 (2001): 206–210.

12. Charles B. Clayman, MD (editor), *The American Medical Association Home Medical Encyclopedia* (New York: Random House, 1989), p. 554.

13. Timothy A. Santongo et al., "Vitamin D Status in Children, Adolescents, and Young Adults with Crohn Disease," *American Journal of Clinical Nutrition* 76 (2002): 1077–1081.

14. John N. Udall Jr., "Crohn's Disease Early in Life and Hypovitaminosis D: Where Do We Go from Here?" *American Journal of Clinical Nutrition* 76 (2002): 909–910.

15. Charles B. Stephensen et al., "Vitamin D Status in Adolescents and Young Adults with HIV Infection," *American Journal of Clinical Nutrition* 83 (2006): 1135–1141.

16. L. Brunvand et al., "Vitamin D Deficiency and Fetal Growth," *Early Human Development* 45, nos. 1–2 (1996): 27–33.

17. L. Brunvand et al., "Congestive Heart Failure Caused by Vitamin D Deficiency," *Acta Pediatrica* 84 (1995): 106–108.

18. Michael F. Holick, PhD, MD, et al., "The Vitamin D Content of Fortified Milk and Infant Formula," *New England Journal of Medicine* 326, no. 18 (1992): 1178–1181.

19. Sulin Cheng et al., "Association of Low 25-Hydroxyvitamin D Concentrations with Elevated Parathryroid Hormone Concentrations and Low Cortical Bone Density in Early Pubertal and Pre-pubertal Finnish Girls," *American Journal of Clinical Nutrition* 78 (2003): 485–492.

Chapter 5

1. Reinhold Vieth et al., "The Urgent Need to Recommend an Intake of Vitamin D that Is Effective," *American Journal of Clinical Nutrition* 85 (2007): 649–650.

2. Heike A. Bischoff-Ferrari et al., "Estimation of Optimal Serum Concentration of 25-Hydroxyvitamin D for Multiple Health Outcomes," *American Journal of Clinical Nutrition* 84 (2006): 18–28.

3. J. N. Hathcock et al., "Risk Assessment for Vitamin D," *American Journal of Clinical Nutrition* 85 (2007): 6–18.

4. Paul F. Jacques et al., "Plasma 25-Hydroxyvitamin D and Its Determinants in an Elderly Population Sample," *American Journal of Clinical Nutrition* 66 (1997): 929–936.

5. J. L. Omdahl et al., "Nutritional Status in a Healthy Elderly Population: Vitamin D," *American Journal of Clinical Nutrition* 36 (1982): 1125–1133.

6. A. R. Webb et al., "An Evaluation of the Relative Contribution of Exposure to Sunlight and of Diet to the Circulating Concentrations of 25-Hydroxyvitamin D in an Elderly Nursing Home Population in Boston," *American Journal of Clinical Nutrition* 51 (1990): 1075–1081.

7. Eric Nagourney, "Shortage of Vitamin D May Weaken the Elderly," *New York Times* (May 1, 2007): F6.

8. A. Heike et al., "Effects of Vitamin D and Calcium Supplementation on Falls: A Randomized Controlled Trial," *Journal of Bone and Mineral Research* 18 (2003): 343–351.

9. Marie C. Chapuy, PhD, et al., "Vitamin D and Calcium to Prevent Hip Fractures in Elderly Women," *New England Journal of Medicine* 32 (1992): 1637–1642.

10. Robert P. Heaney, MD, "Hip Fracture: A Nutritional Perspective," *Proceedings for the Society of Experimental Biology and Medicine* 200 (1992): 153–156.

11. "Lead, Vitamin C, Vitamin D, and Iron," *American Journal of Epidemiology* 147 (1998): 1162–1174.

12. T. Diamond et al., "Hip Fractures in Elderly Men: The Importance of Sub-Clinical Vitamin D Deficiency and Hypogonadism," *Medical Journal of Australia* 169 (August 3, 1998): 138–141.

13. J. Heller, "The Vitamin Status and Its Adequacy in the Elderly: An International Overview," *International Journal of Vitamin and Nutritional Research* 69, no. 3 (1999): 160–168.

14. R. D. Semba et al., "Vitamin D Deficiency among Older Women with and without Disability," *American Journal of Clinical Nutrition* 72 (2000): 1529–1534.

15. F. Michael Gloth III, MD, et al., "Vitamin D Deficiency in Housebound Elderly Persons," *JAMA* 274, no. 21 (1995): 1683–1686.

16. M. McKenna, "Differences in Vitamin D Status between Countries in Young Adults and the Elderly," *American Journal of Medicine* 93 (1992): 69–77.

17. Norman H. Bell, "Editorial: Vitamin D Metabolism, Aging and Bone Loss," *Journal of Clinical Endocrinology and Metabolism* 80, no. 4 (1995): 1051ff.

18. K. Schumann, "Interactions between Drugs and Vitamins at Advanced Age," *International Journal of Vitamin and Nutrition Research* 69, no. 3 (1999): 173–178.

19. Marie C. Chapuy, PhD, et al., "Effect of Calcium and Cholecalciferol Treatment for Three Years on Hip Fractures in Elderly Women," *British Medical Journal* 308 (April 23, 1994): 1081–1082.

20. Ailsa Goulding, PhD, "Lightening the Fracture Load: Growing Evidence Suggests Many Older New Zealanders Would Benefit from More Vitamin D," *New Zealand Medical Journal* 112 (September 10, 1999): 329–330.

21. Joseph R. Sharkey et al., "Summary Measure of Dietary Muscoloskeletal Nutrient (Calcium, Vitamin D, Magnesium, and Phosphorus) Intakes Are Associated with Lower Extremity Physical Performance in Homebound Elderly Men and Women," *American Journal of Clinical Nutrition* 77 (2003): 847–856.

22. Rob M. van Dam et al., "Potentially Modifiable Determinants of Vitamin D Status in an Older Population in the Netherlands: The Hoorn Study," *American Journal of Clinical Nutrition* 85 (2007): 755–761.

23. E. Hypponen et al., "Hypervitaminosis D in British Adults at Age 45: Nationwide Cohort Study of Dietary and Lifestyle Predictors," *American Journal of Clinical Nutrition* 85 (2007): 860–868.

24. R. L. Prince et al., "Effects of Ergocalciferol Added to Calcium on the Risk of Falls in Elderly High-Risk Women," *Archives of Internal Medicine* 168, no. 1 (2008): 103–108.

Chapter 6

1. Charles B. Clayman, MD (editor), *The American Medical Association Home Medical Encyclopedia* (New York: Random House, 1989), pp. 192ff.

2. Ego Seeman, MD, and Pierre D. Delmas, MD, "Bone Quality—The Material and Structural Basis of Bone Strength and Fragility," *New England Journal of Medicine* 354 (May 25, 2006): 2250–2261.

3. Heike A. Bischoff-Ferrari, MD, MPH, et al., "Fracture Prevention with Vitamin D Supplements," *JAMA* 293, no. 18 (2005): 2257–2264.

4. Nicholas Bakalar, "Older Bones See Benefit of Calcium and Vitamin D," *New York Times* (September 4, 2007): F6.

5. Anne M. Wolff, RD, and Andrew Wolff, MD, "Evidence Based Use of Vitamin and Mineral Supplementation," *Hospital Medicine* (December 1998): 53–54.

6. R. Deroisy et al., "Effect of Two 1-Year Calcium and Vitamin D$_3$ Treatments on Bone Remodeling Markers and Femoral Bone Density in Elderly Women," *Current Therapeutic Research* 59, no. 12 (December 1998): 850–862.

7. Jean-Philippe Bonjour, MD, et al., "Nutritional Aspects of Hip Fractures," *Bone* 18, no. 3 (March 1996): 139S–144S.

8. K. E. Wical and P. Brussee, "Effect of Calcium and Vitamin D Supplement on Alveolar Ridge Resorption in Denture Patients," *Journal of Prosthetic Dentistry* 41, no. 1 (January 1979): 4–11.

9. Bess Dawson-Hughes, MD, et al., "Effect of Calcium and Vitamin D Supplementation on Bone Density in Men and Women 65 Years of Age or Older," *New England Journal of Medicine* 337, no. 10 (1997): 670–676.

10. Bess Dawson-Hughes, MD, and Susan S. Harris, "Calcium Intake Influences the Association of Protein Intake with Rates of Bone Loss in Elderly Men and Women," *American Journal of Clinical Nutrition* 75 (2002): 773–779.

11. R. D. Jackson et al., "Calcium Plus Vitamin D Supplementation and the Risk of Fractures," *New England Journal of Medicine* 354 (2006): 669–683.

12. Susan Terris, MD, PhD, "Calcium plus Vitamin D and the Risk of Hip Fractures," *New England Journal of Medicine* 354, no. 21 (2006): 2285.

13. Gerson T. Lesser, MD, *New England Journal of Medicine* 354, no. 21 (2006): 2285–2286.

14. Bess Dawson-Hughes, MD, *New England Journal of Medicine* 354, no. 21 (2006): 2286.

Chapter 7

1. Charles B. Clayman, MD (editor), *The American Medical Association Home Medical Encyclopedia* (New York: Random House, 1989), p. 696.

2. Mark A. Stevens (editor), *Merriam-Webster's Collegiate Encyclopedia* (Springfield, Mass.: Merriam-Webster, Inc., 2000), p. 638.

3. Yoshihiro Sato et al., "Hypovitaminosis D and Decreased Bone Mineral Density in Amyotrophic Lateral Sclerosis," *European Neurology* 37 (1997): 225–229.

4. Geoffrey Dean, MD, "ALS: Patterns and Progress," *Medical and Health Annual* (Chicago: Encyclopaedia Britannica, Inc., 1995), pp. 364ff.

5. Robert A. Ronzio, PhD, *The Encyclopedia of Nutrition and Good Health* (New York: Facts on File, Inc., 1997), p. 17.

6. R. Bruce Martin, "Aluminum: A Neurotoxic Product of Acid Rain," *Accounts of Chemical Research* 27 (1994): 204–210.

7. G. B. van der Voet and F. A. Wolff, "Intestinal Absorption of Aluminum: Effect of Sodium and Calcium," *Archives of Toxicology* 72 (1998): 110–114.

Chapter 8

1. Mukti H. Sarma, PhD, "Cancer," *Medical and Health Annual* (Chicago: Encyclopaedia Britannica, Inc., 1994), pp. 250ff.

2. A. Ensminger et al., *Foods & Nutrition Encyclopedia.* (Clovis, CA: Pegus Press, 1983), pp. 316ff.

3. Florence Rozen et al., "Antiproliferative Action of Vitamin D Related Compounds and Insulin Like Growth Factor Binding Protein 5 Accumulation," *Journal of the National Cancer Institute* 89, no. 9 (May 7, 1997): 652–656.

4. Joan M. Lappe et al., "Vitamin D and Calcium Supplementation Reduces Cancer Risk: Results of a Randomized Trial," *American Journal of Clinical Nutrition* 85 (2007): 1586–1591.

5. George P. Studzinski and Dorothy C. Moore, "Sunlight: Can't It Prevent as Well as Cause Cancer?" *Cancer Research* 55 (September 15, 1995): 4014–4022.

6. Bill Sardi, "Vitamin D Is for Cancer Defense," *Nutrition Science News* 5, no. 3 (March 2000): 100–102.

7. Faye B. Bass, MS, et al., "The Need for Dietary Counseling of Cancer Patients as Indicated by Nutrient and Supplement Intake," *Journal of the American Dietetic Association* (1995): 1319–1321.

8. L. Magrassi et al., "Effects of Vitamin D and Retinoic Acid on Human Glioblastoma Cell Lines," *Acta Neurochirurgica* 133 (1995): 184–190.

9. J. A. Knight et al., "Vitamin D and Reduced Risk of Breast Cancer: A Population Based Case Control Study," *Cancer Epidemiology Biomarkers and Prevention* 16, no. 3 (2007): 422–429.

10. "Children's Health," *Health Gems* 7, no. 1 (2006): 10.

11. K. Carroll et al., "Calcium and Carcinogenesis of the Mammary Gland," *American Journal of Clinical Nutrition* 54 (1991): 206S–208S.

12. E. M. John et al., "Vitamin D and Breast Cancer Risk: The NHANES I Epidemiologic Follow-Up Study: 1971–1975 to 1992," *Cancer Epidemiology, Biomarkers and Prevention* 8 (1999): 399–406.

13. James E. Marti, *Alternative Health & Medicine Encyclopedia* (Detroit: Visible Ink Press, 1995), p. 52.

14. Susan S. Tomlinson, "Dietary and Lifestyle Factors Associated with Breast Cancer Risk," *Journal of the American Academy of Physician Assistants* 7 (1994): 622–634.

15. J. van Leeuwen et al. "Vitamin D and Breast Cancer," *Physiology, Molecular Biology, and Clinical Applications* 24 (1999): 411–429.

16. M. Lipkin and H. L. Newmark, "Vitamin D, Calcium and Prevention of Breast Cancer: A Review," *Journal of the American College of Nutrition* 18, no. 5 (1999): 392S–397S.

17. "Diet of Young Girls May Increase Their Risk of Breast Cancer: Inadequate Levels of Dietary Calcium and Vitamin D May Increase the Risk of Breast and Other Cancers for Young Females and the Elderly," *Primary Care and Cancer* 14, no. 2 (February 1994): 8.

18. Roberd H. Bostick et al., "Relation of Calcium, Vitamin D, and Dairy Food Intake to Incidence of Colon Cancer among Older Women: The Iowa Woman's Health Study," *American Journal of Epidemiology* 137, no. 2 (1993): 1302–1317.

19. E. Oh et al., "Calcium and Vitamin D Intakes in Relation to Risk of Distal Colorectal Adenoma in Women," *American Journal of Epidemiology* 165, no. 10 (March 22, 2007): 1178–1186.

20. Marcus J. Burnstein, MD, "Dietary Factors Related to Colorectal Neoplasms," *Colorectal Cancer* 73, no. 1 (February 1993): 13–29.

21. James C. Fleet, "Dairy Consumption and the Prevention of Colon Cancer: Is There More to the Story than Calcium?" *American Journal of Clinical Nutrition* 83 (2006): 527–528.

22. Jeffrey A. Meyerhardt, MD, et al., "Association of Dietary Factors with Cancer Recurrence and Survival in Patients with Stage III Colon Cancer," *JAMA* 298, no. 7 (2007): 754–764.

23. J. Wactawski-Wende, PhD, et al., "Calcium plus Vitamin D Supplementation and the Risk of Colorectal Cancer," *New England Journal of Medicine* 354 (2006): 1102.

24. Michael F. Holick, MD, PhD, "Calcium plus Vitamin D and the Risk of Colorectal Cancer," *New England Journal of Medicine* 354, no. 21 (2006): 2287.

25. Edward Giovannucci, MD, ScD, *New England Journal of Medicine,* 354, no. 21 (2006): 2287–2288.

26. Jean Wactawski-Wende, PhD, et al., *New England Journal of Medicine,* 354, no. 21 (2006): 2288.

27. Roger Bouillon, MD, PhD, et al., "Vitamin D Deficiency," *New England Journal of Medicine* 357, no. 19 (2007): 1980.

28. Robert C. Cava, MD, and Andrei Nicole D. Javier, *New England Journal of Medicine* 357, no. 19 (2007): 1981.

29. William R. Howe, MD, and Robert Dellavalle, MD, PhD, *New England Journal of Medicine* 357, no. 19 (2007): 1981.

30. Giampiero Igli Baroncelli, MD, *New England Journal of Medicine* 357, no. 19 (2007): 1981.

31. Michael F. Holick, MD, PhD *New England Journal of Medicine* 357, no. 19 (2007): 1981–1982.

32. E. Lefkowitz and C. Garland, "Sunlight, Vitamin D and Ovarian Cancer Mortality Rates in U.S. Women," *International Journal of Epidemiology* 23, no. 6 (1994): 1133–1136.

33. Nicholas Bakalar, "Vitamin D Is Said to Cut Pancreatic Cancer Risk," *New York Times* (September 19, 2006): F6.

34. Nicholas Bakalar, "Sun May Lower Risk of Endometrial Cancer," *New York Times* (November 27, 2007): F6.

Chapter 9

1. "Heart Disease and Stroke Statistical Update," *American Heart Association,* Dallas, Texas, 2006.

2. Kirk Hamilton, "Coronary Artery/Heart Disease, Cholesterol and Sunlight," *Clinical Pearls* (Sacramento: IT Services, 1997), pp. 298–299. *Also,* David S. Grimes, MD, "Sunlight, Cholesterol and Coronary Heart Disease," *Quarterly Journal of Medicine* 89 (1996): 579–589.

3. J. P. Forman et al., "Plasma 25-Hydroxyvitamin D Levels and Risk of Incident Hypertension," *Hypertension* 49 (March 19, 2007): 1063–1069.

4. Karol E. Watson, MD, et al., "Active Serum Vitamin D Levels Are Inversely Correlated with Coronary Calcification," *Circulation* 96 (1997): 1755–1760.

5. Elizabeth Shane, MD, et al., "Bone Mass, Vitamin D Deficiency, and Hyperparathyroidism in Congestive Heart Failure," *American Journal of Medicine* 103 (1997): 197–207.

6. D. Martins et al., "Prevalence of Cardiovascular Risk Factors and the Serum Levels of 25-Hydroxyvitamin D in the United States: Data from the Third National Health and Nutrition Examination Survey," *Archives of Internal Medicine* 167 (2007): 1159–1165.

7. A. Zitterman et al., "Low Vitamin D Status: A Contributing Factor in the Pathogenesis of Congestive Heart Failure," *Journal of the American College of Cardiology* 41, no. 1 (2003): 105–112.

8. L. Brunvand et al., "Congestive Heart Failure Caused by Vitamin D Deficiency," *Acta Pediatrica* 84 (1995): 106–108.

9. P. G. Avery et al., "Cardiac Failure Due to Hypercalcemia of Nutritional Osteomalacia," *European Heart Journal* 13 (1992): 426–427.

10. Mike Mitka, "Vitamin D Deficits May Affect Heart Health," *JAMA* 299, no. 7 (February 20, 2008): 753.

11. Suzanne E. Judd et al., "Optimal Vitamin D Status Attenuates the Age-Associated Increase in Systolic Blood Pressure in White Americans: Results from the Third National Heath and Nutrition Examination Survey," *American Journal of Clinical Nutrition* 87 (January 2008): 136–141.

Chapter 10

1. Charles B. Clayman, MD (editor), *The American Medical Association Home Medical Encyclopedia* (New York: Random House, 1989), p. 245.

2. Peter H. R. Green, MD, and Christophe Cellier, MD, PhD "Celiac Disease," *New England Journal of Medicine* 357 (October 25, 2007): 1731–1743.

3. Seymour Mishkin, MD, "Effects of Dietary Treatment on Bone Mineral Density in Celiac Disease," *Nutrition & the M.D.* 25, no. 1 (January 2000): 6–7.

4. Carlos Mautalen, MD, et al., "Effect of Treatment on Bone Mass: Mineral Metabolism, and Body Composition in Untreated Celiac Disease Patients," *American Journal of Gastroenterology* 92, no. 2 (February 1997): 313–318.

5. A. Pini et al., "Muscular Disorders in Celiac Disease," *Epilepsy and Other Neurological Disorders in Coeliac Disease* 41 (1997): 301–303.

6. Lucia J. Chartrand, RD, et al., "Wheat Starch into Tolerance in Patients with Celiac Disease," *Journal of the American Dietetic Association* 97, no. 6 (June 1997): 612–618.

7. Aldo Bertoli et al., "A Woman with Bone Pain, Fractures, and Malabsorption," *The Lancet* 347 (February 3, 1996): 300.

8. Jacques Schmitz, MD, "Lack of Oats Toxicity in Celiac Disease," *British Medical Journal* 314 (January 18, 1997): 159–160.

9. G. L. de Angelis et al., "Neurological Findings in Adults with Unknown Celiac Disease," *Epilepsy and Other Neurological Disorders in Celiac Disease* 16 (1998): 342–344.

10. Tricia Thompson, RD, "Do Oats Belong in a Gluten-Free Diet?" *Journal of the American Dietetic Association* 97 (1997): 1413–1416.

11. Stefano Mora et al., "Effect of Gluten Free Diet on Bone Mineral Content in Growing Patients with Celiac Disease," *American Journal of Clinical Nutrition* 57 (1993): 224–228.

12. Peter Howdle, MD, "Why Lifelong Diet Matters in Celiac Disease," *The Practitioner* 238 (1994): 687–691.

Chapter 11

1. Charles B. Clayman, MD (editor), *The American Medical Association Home Medical Encyclopedia* (New York: Random House, 1989), p. 320.

2. R. H. Driscoll Jr. et al., "Vitamin D Deficiency and Bone Disease in Patients with Crohn's Disease," *Gastroenterology* 83 (December 1982): 1252–1258.

3. H. Vogelsang et al., "Prevention of Bone Mineral Loss in Patients with Crohn's Disease by Long-Term Oral Vitamin D Supplementation," *European Journal of Gastroenterology and Hepatology* 7, no. 7 (July 1995): 609–614.

4. G. A. Leichtmann et al., "Internal Absorption of Cholecalciferol and 25-Hydrocycholecalciferol in Patients with both Crohn's Disease and Internal Resection," *American Journal of Clinical Nutrition* 54 (1991): 548–552.

5. Donald F. Tarpley, MD, et al., editors, *The Columbia University College of Physicians and Surgeons Complete Home Medical Guide* (New York: Crown Publishers, Inc., 1985), p. 530.

6. A. D. Harries et al., "Vitamin D Status in Crohn's Disease: Association with Nutrition and Disease Activity," *Gut* 26 (1985): 1197–1203.

7. Peggy Peck, "Vitamin Supplements Critical to All Inflammatory Bowel Disease Patients," *Family Practice News* (May 15, 1994): 4.

8. Michael T. Murray, ND, *Natural Alternatives to Over the Counter and Prescription Drugs* (New York: William Morrow and Co., Inc., 1994), pp. 157–158.

9. Daniel K. Podolsky, MD, et al., "Case 8-2006: A 71 Year Old Man with Crohn's Disease and Altered Mental Status," *New England Journal of Medicine* 354 (2006): 1178–1184.

10. Charles B. Clayman, MD (editor), *AMA Home Medical Encyclopedia,* p. 657.

Chapter 12

1. Charles B. Clayman, MD (editor), *The American Medical Association Home Medical Encyclopedia* (New York: Random House, 1989), p. 328.

2. Anne Stephenson et al., "Cholecalciferol Significantly Increases 25-Hydroxyvitamin D Concentrations in Adults with Cystic Fibrosis," *American Journal of Clinical Nutrition* 85 (2007): 1307–1311.

3. Rosemary J. Rayner, "Fat Soluble Vitamins in Cystic Fibrosis," *Proceedings of the Nutrition Society* 51 (1992): 245–250.

4. Siobhan Carr, MD, et al., "The Role of Vitamins in Cystic Fibrosis," *Journal of the Royal Society,* Med 93, Suppl. 38 (2000): 14–19.

5. Richard C. Henderson, MD, PhD, and Gayle Lester, MD "Vitamin D Levels in Children with Cystic Fibrosis," *Southern Medical Journal* 90, no. 4 (April 1997): 378–382.

6. Michael P. Boyle, MD, "Adult Cystic Fibrosis," *JAMA* 298, no. 15 (October 17, 2007): 1787–1793.

7. Alisha J. Rovner et al., "Vitamin D Insufficiency in Children, Adolescents, and Young Adults with Cystic Fibrosis despite Routine Oral Supplementation," *American Journal of Clinical Nutrition* 86 (2007): 1694–1699.

Chapter 13

1. American Diabetes Association, Atlanta, Georgia. Various publications, 2007.

2. Charles B. Clayman, MD (editor), *The American Medical Association Home Medical Encyclopedia* (New York: Random House, 1989), pp. 349ff.

3. Tracy Hampton, PhD, "Studies Probe Value of Lifestyle Changes for Preventing Type 2 Diabetes," *JAMA* 298, no. 6 (August 8, 2007): 617.

4. Elsa S. Strotmeyer, PhD, et al., "Middle Aged Pre-menopausal Women with Type 1 Diabetes Have Lower Bone Mineral Density and Calcaneal Quantitative Ultrasound than Non-Diabetic Women," *Diabetes Care* 29 (2006): 306–311.

5. Earl S. Ford, MD, MPH, et al., "Concentrations of Serum Vitamin D and the Metabolic Syndrome among U.S. Adults," *Diabetes Care* 28 (2005): 1228–1229.

6. Massimo Cigolini, MD, et al., "Serum 25-Hydroxyvitamin D_3 Concentrations and Prevalence of Cardiovascular Disease among Type 2 Diabetic Patients," *Diabetes Care* 29 (2006): 722–724.

7. David J. Di Cesar et al., "Vitamin D Deficiency Is More Common in Type 2 than in Type 1 Diabetes," *Diabetes Care* 29 (2006): 174.

8. R. Scragg et al., "Serum 25-Hydroxyvitamin D₃ Levels Decreased in Impaired Glucose Tolerance and Diabetes," *Diabetes Research and Clinical Practice* 27, no. 3 (1995): 181–188.

9. G. Dahlquist et al., "Vitamin D Supplement in Early Childhood and Risk of Type 1 (Insulin-Dependent) Diabetes Mellitus," *Diabetologia* 42 (1999): 51–54.

10. K. C. R. Baynes et al., "Vitamin D Glucose Tolerance and Insulinemia in Elderly Men," *Diabetologia* 40 (1997): 344–347.

11. O. Vaarala et al., "Environmental Factors in the Aetiology of Childhood Diabetes," *Diabetes and Nutrition Metabolism* 12, no. 2 (1999): 75–85.

12. Maria Thomas and Loren W. Greene, MD, *The Unofficial Guide to Living with Diabetes* (New York: Macmillan, 1999), pp. 103–104.

13. Kirk Hamilton, "Glucose Tolerance, Insulinemia and Vitamin D," *Clinical Pearls* (Sacramento: IT Services, Inc., 1997), p. 305. *Also,* B. J. Boucher, MD, "Vitamin D, Glucose Tolerance and Insulinemia in Elderly Men," *Diabetologia* 40 (1997): 344–347.

14. Anastassios G. Pittas, MD, et al., "Vitamin D and Calcium Intake in Relation to Type 2 Diabetes in Women," *Diabetes Care* 29, no. 3 (2006): 650–656.

15. Lars C. Stene et al., "Use of Cod Liver Oil during the First Year of Life Is Associated with Lower Risk of Childhood Onset Type Diabetes: A Large, Population Based, Case Control Study," *American Journal of Clinical Nutrition* 78 (2003): 1128–1134.

16. Stefanie S. Schleithoff et al., "Vitamin D Supplementation Improves Cytokine Profiles in Patients with Congestive Heart Failure: A Double Blind, Randomized, Placebo Controlled Trial," *American Journal of Clinical Nutrition* 83 (2006): 754–759.

17. Reinhold Vieth, PhD, and Samantha Kimball, "Vitamin D in Congestive Heart Failure." *American Journal of Clinical Nutrition* 83 (2006): 731–732.

18. Robert P. Heaney, MD, et al., "Human Serum 25-Hydroxycholecalciferol Response to Extended Oral Dosing with Cholecalciferol," *American Journal of Clinical Nutrition* 77 (2003): 204–210.

Chapter 14

1. Randolph Lee Clark, MD, and Russell W. Cumley, PhD, *The Book of Health* (New York: Van Nostrand Reinhold Co., 1973), p. 419.

2. Donald F. Tapley, MD, et al., medical editors, *The Columbia University College of Physicians and Surgeons Complete Home Medical Guide* (New York: Crown Publishers, Inc., 1985), pp. 699–700.

3. Thomas Dietrich et al., "Association between Serum Concentrations of 25-Hydroxyvitamin D and Gingival Inflammation," *American Journal of Clinical Nutrition* 82 (2005): 575–580.

4. Thomas Dietrich et al., "Association between Serum Concentrations of 25-Hydroxyvitamin D₃ and Periodontal Disease in the U.S. Population," *American Journal of Clinical Nutrition* 80 (2004): 108–113.

Chapter 15

1. Robert A. Ronzio, PhD, *The Encyclopedia of Nutrition and Good Health* (New York: Facts on File, Inc., 1997), pp. 243–244.

2. Ilkka Laaksi et al., "An Association of Serum Vitamin D Concentrations—Less than 40 nmol/l with Acute Respiratory Tract Infection in Young Finnish Men," *American Journal of Clinical Nutrition* 86 (2007): 714–717.

3. Kirk Hamilton, "Vitamin D Deficiency in the Elderly," *The Experts Speak* (Sacramento: IT Services, 1996), pp. 203–204. *Also,* F. Michael Gloth III, MD, "Vitamin D Deficiency in Older People," *Journal of the American Geriatric Society* 43:822-828, 1995.

4. K. Z. Long and J. L. Santos, "Vitamins and the Regulation of the Immune Response," *Pediatric Infectious Disease Journal* 18 no. 3 (March 1999): 283–290.

5. John E. Morley, MB, "Nutritional Modulation of Behavior and Immunocompetence," *Nutrition Reviews* 52, no. 8 (1994): S6–S8.

6. Kirk Hamilton, "Autoimmune Disease and Vitamin D," *Clinical Pearls* (Sacramento: IT Services, 2000), p. 78. *Also,* Margherita T. Cantorna, PhD, "Vitamin D and Autoimmunity: Is Vitamin D Status an Environmental Factor Affecting Autoimmune Disease Prevalence," *Proceedings of the Society for Experimental Biology and Medicine* 223 (2000): 230–233.

Chapter 16

1. Randolph Lee Clark, MD, and Russell W. Cumley, PhD, *The Book of Health* (New York: Van Nostrand Reinhold Co., 1979), pp. 385, 598, 633.

2. Geoffrey Dean, MD, "Multiple Sclerosis," *Medical and Health Annual* (Chicago: Encyclopaedia Britannica, Inc., 1994), pp. 363ff.

3. Kassandra L. Munger, MSc, et al., "Serum 25-Hydroxyvitamin D Levels and Risk of Multiple Sclerosis," *JAMA* 296 (2006): 2832–2838.

4. Colleen E. Hayes et al., "Vitamin D and Multiple Sclerosis," *Proceedings of the Society of Experimental Biology and Medicine* 216 (1997): 21–27.

5. Samantha M. Kimball et al., "Safety of Vitamin D₃ in Adults with Multiple Sclerosis," *American Journal of Clinical Nutrition* 86 (2007): 645–651.

6. Jeri Nieves, PhD, et al., "High Prevalence of Vitamin D Deficiency and Reduced Bone Mass in Multiple Sclerosis," *Neurology* 44 (September 1994): 1687.

7. G. Dick, "Natural History of Multiple Sclerosis," *Journal of the Royal Society of Medicine* 85 (July 1992): 824–825.

8. R. A. Hughes, "Pathogenesis of Multiple Sclerosis," *Journal of the Royal Society of Medicine* 85 (July 1992): 373–376.

9. D. Shabas et al., "Preventive Healthcare in Women with Multiple Sclerosis," *Journal of Women's Health & Gender-Based Medicine* 9, no. 4 (May 2000): 389–395.

10. Gary G. Schwartz, PhD, MPH, "Multiple Sclerosis and Prostate Cancer," *Neuroepidemiology* 11 (1992): 244–254.

11. Gary G. Schwartz, PhD, MPH, "Hypothesis: Calcitriol Mediates Pregnancy's Protective Effect on Multiple Sclerosis," *Archives of Neurology* 50 (May 1993): 455.

Chapter 17

1. Charles B. Clayman, MD (editor), *The American Medical Association Home Guide* (New York: Random House, 1989), p. 753.

2. Randolph Lee Clark, MD, and Russell W. Cumley, PhD, *The Book of Health* (New York: Van Nostrand Reinhold Co., 1973), p. 301.

3. T. E. McAlindon et al., "Relation of Dietary Intake and Serum Levels of Vitamin D in Progression of Osteoarthritis of the Knee among Participants in the Framingham Study," *Annals of Internal Medicine* 125, no. 5 (1996): 353–359.

4. Marc K. Effron, MD, "Cardiovascular Disease," *Medical and Health Annual* (Chicago: Encyclopaedia Britannica, Inc., 1995), p. 242.

5. T. E. McAlindon, "Osteoarthritis: Role of Nutrition and Dietary Supplement Intervention," *Primary and Secondary Preventive Nutrition* 17 (2000): 291–305.

6. N. E. Lane et al., "Serum Vitamin D Levels and Incident Changes of Radiographic Hip Osteoarthritis: A Longitudinal Study," *Arthritis and Rheumatism* 42, no. 5 (May 1999): 854–860.

7. T. E. McAlindon, "Can Diet Affect the Risk and Progression of Osteoarthritis? Studies of Obesity, Folate, and Vitamins C, E, and D," *Women's Health in Primary Care* 3, no. 10 (2000): 741–747.

8. "Vitamin D Deficiency Common in Arthritis," *The Nutrition Report* (January 1994): 3.

Chapter 18

1. T. S. Dharmarajan et al., "Vitamin D Deficiency and Osteomalacia in Older Adults," *Family Practice Recertification* 23, no. 5 (2001): 41–50.

2. Charles B. Clayman, MD (editor), *The American Medical Association Home Medical Encyclopedia* (New York: Random House, 1989), p. 755.

3. Reinhold Vieth, "Vitamin D Supplementation, 25-Hydroxyvitamin D Concentrations, and Safety," *American Journal of Clinical Nutrition* 69 (1999): 842–856.

4. A. V. G. Taylor and P. H. Wise, "Treatment of Vitamin D Deficient Osteomalacia May Unmask Autonomous Hyperthyroidism," *British Medical Journal* (1997): 813–815.

Chapter 19

1. "Fast Facts on Osteoporosis," *National Osteoporosis Foundation,* Washington D.C., July 2005.

2. Genell J. Subak-Sharpe (editor), *The Physicians' Manual for Patients* (New York: Times Books, 1984), pp. 98ff.

3. Gina Kolata, "What's Inside Those Old Bones? With Osteoporosis, It Seems to Be Fat," *New York Times* (July 26, 2005): F5.

4. "Osteoporosis Prevention, Diagnosis, and Therapy, NIH Consensus Development Panel on Osteoporosis Prevention, Diagnosis, and Therapy," *JAMA* 285, no. 6 (2001): 785–795.

5. Michael F. Holick, PhD, MD, "Nutrients Critical for Bone Health: Vitamin D," *Paper read at the 21st Annual Public Health Nutrition Update Conference,* William and Ida Friday Continuing Education Center, Chapel Hill, North Carolina, April 12–13, 1995.

6. Isadore Rosenfeld, MD, "Keep Your Bones Strong," *Parade* (October 14, 2007): 10–11.

7. Katherine L. Tucker et al., "Bone Mineral Density and Dietary Patterns in Older Adults: The Framingham Osteoporosis Study," *American Journal of Clinical Nutrition* 76 (2002): 245–252.

8. Pierre J. Meunier, "Calcium, Vitamin D and Vitamin K in the Prevention of Fractures Due to Osteoporosis," *Osteoporos International* 2 (1999): S48–S52.

9. M. Tilyard et al., "Treatment of Postmenopausal Osteoporosis with Calcitriol or Calcium," *New England Journal of Medicine* 326 (1992): 357–362.

10. Ian R. Reid, MD, "Therapy of Osteoporosis: Calcium, Vitamin D, and Exercise," *American Journal of the Medical Sciences* 312, no. 6 (1996): 278–286.

11. Richard L. Prince, MD, "Diet and the Prevention of Osteoporotic Fractures," *New England Journal of Medicine* 337 (1997): 701–702.

12. Philip Sambrook, MD, et al., "Prevention of Corticosteroid Osteoporosis: A Comparison of Calcium, Calcitriol, and Calcitonin," *New England Journal of Medicine* 328, nos. 2–4 (1993): 1747–1752.

13. Peter R. Ebeling, MD, "Osteoporosis in Men," *New England Journal of Medicine* 358 (2008): 1472–1482.

Chapter 20

1. Charles B. Clayman, MD (editor), *The American Medical Association Home Medical Encyclopedia* (New York: Random House, 1989), pp. 825–826.

2. Michael F. Holick, MD, PhD "Vitamin D Deficiency," *New England Journal of Medicine* 357, no. 3 (July 19, 2007): 266–281.

3. Elizabeth H. Corder et al., "Seasonal Variation in Vitamin D, Vitamin D Binding Proteins and Dehydroepiandrosterone: Risk of Prostate Cancer in Black and White Men," *Cancer Epidemiology, Biomarkers and Prevention* 4 (September 1995): 655–659.

4. Ronald K. Ross, MD, and Brian E. Henderson, "Do Diet and Androgens Alter Prostate Cancer Risk via a Common Etiology Pathway?" *Journal of the National Cancer Institute* 86, no. 4 (February 16, 1994): 252–255.

5. "Prostate Cancer and Vitamin D," *Cancer Research* 55 (1996): 4108–4110.

6. Robert C. Atkins, MD, *Dr. Atkins' Vita-Nutrient Solution* (New York: Simon & Schuster, 1998), p. 106.

7. Gary G. Schwartz, PhD, "Multiple Sclerosis and Prostate Cancer: What Do Their Similar Geographies Suggest?" *Neuroepidemiology* 11 (1992): 244–254.

8. Peter T. Scardino, MD, and Judith Kelman, *Dr. Peter Scardino's Prostate Book* (New York: Avery/Penguin Group, 2006), pp. 127–128.

9. D. M. Peehl et al., "Vitamin D and Prostate Cancer," *Journal of Endocrinology Investigation* 17, Suppl. 1–3 (1994).

10. Gregory Maltz, "Sunlight May Protect against Cancers and Melanoma," *Family Practice News* (February 1, 1996): 21.

11. J. P. Bonjour et al., "Calcium Intake and Vitamin D Metabolism and Action, in Healthy Conditions and in Prostate Cancer," *British Journal of Nutrition* 97, no. 4 (2007): 596–597.

Chapter 21

1. A. Ensminger et al., *Foods & Nutrition Encyclopedia* (Clovis, CA: Pegus Press, 1983), pp. 1943ff.

2. A. Mustafa et al., "Dilated Cardiomyopathy as a First Sign of Nutritional Vitamin D Deficiency: Rickets in Infancy," *Canadian Journal of Cardiology* 15, no. 6 (June 1999): 699–701.

3. Joseph H. Clark, MD, et al., "Symptomatic Vitamin A and D Deficiencies in an Eight Year Old with Autism," *Journal of Parenteral and Enteral Nutrition* 17, no. 3 (May–June 1993): 284–286.

4. B. A. Wharton, "Low Plasma Vitamin D in Asian Toddlers in Britain," *British Medical Journal* 318 (January 2, 1999): 2–3.

5. Binita R. Shah, MD, and Laurence Finberg, MD, "Single-Day Therapy for Nutritional D Deficiency Rickets: A Preferred Method," *Journal of Pediatrics* 125, no. 3 (September 1994): 487–490.

6. Gulam Nabi, MD, "Vitamin D Deficiency Rickets in Riyadh," *Annals of Saudi Medicine* 12, no. 1 (1992): 108–109.

7. Hussein Salman, MD, *Annals of Saudi Medicine* 12, no. 1 (1992): 109.

Chapter 22

1. Randolph Lee Clark, MD, and Russell W. Cumley, PhD, *The Book of Health* (New York: Van Nostrand Reinhold Co., 1973), pp. 229ff.

2. Genell J. Subak-Sharpe (editor), *The Physicians' Manual for Patients* (New York: Times Books, 1984), pp. 338–340.

3. J. F. Bourke et al., "Vitamin D Analogues in Psoriasis: Effects on Systemic Calcium Homeostatis," *British Journal of Dermatology* 135 (1996): 347–354.

4. S. Takamoto et al., "Effect of 1-Alpha-Hydroxycholecalciferon on Psoriasis Vulgaris: A Pilot Study," *Calcified Tissue International* 39, no. 6 (December 1986): 360–364.

5. S. Morimoto et al., "Topical Administration of 1,25-Dihydroxyvitamin D_3 for Psoriasis: Report of 5 Cases," *Calcified Tissue International* 38, no. 2 (February 1986): 119–122.

6. Luigi Naldi, MD, "Dietary Factors and the Risk of Psoriasis: Results of an Italian Case Control Study," *British Journal of Dermatology* 134 (1996): 101–106.

7. M. Gerritsen et al., "Topical Treatment of Psoriatic Plaque with 1,25-Dihydroxyvitamin D₃: A Cell Biological Study," *British Journal of Dermatology* 128 (1993): 666–673.

8. H. Sacki et al., "Polymorphisms of Vitamin D Receptor Gene in Japanese Patients with Psoriasis Vulgari," *Journal of Dermatological Science* 30, no. 2 (2002): 167–171.

9. A. Perez et al., "Safety and Efficacy of Oral Calcitriol (1,25-Dihydroxyvitamin D₃) for the Treatment of Psoriasis," *British Journal of Dermatology* 134 (1996): 1070–1078.

10. J. Barth-Jones and P. H. Hutchinson, "Vitamin D Analogues and Psoriasis," *British Journal of Dermatology* 127 (1992): 71–78.

11. K. Kragballe, MD, "Vitamin D Analogues in the Treatment of Psoriasis," *Journal of Cellular Biochemistry* 49 (1992): 46–52.

12. Petra Milde, MD, "Vitamin D: New Aspects and Perspectives," *Hautarzt* 42 (1991): 671–676.

13. Donald F. Tapley, MD, et al., editors, *The Columbia University College of Physicians and Surgeons Complete Home Medical Guide* (New York: Crown Publishers, Inc., 1985), pp. 584–585.

14. Alice Feinstein (editor), *Prevention's Healing with Vitamins* (Emmaus, PA: Rodale Press, Inc., 1996), pp. 496ff.

15. P. G. Humbert et al., "Localized Scleroderma Response to 1,25-Dihydroxyvitamin D₃," *Clinical and Experimental Dermatology* 159, no. 5 (September 1990): 396–398.

16. P. G. Humbert et al., "Treatment of Scleroderma with Oral 1,25-Dihydroxyvitamin D₃: Evaluation of Skin Involvement Using Non-Invasive Techniques. Results of an Open Prospective Trial," *Acta Derm. Venerol. (Stockholm)* 73 (1993): 449–451.

17. L. Y. Matauoka et al., "Cutaneous Vitamin D₃ Formation in Progressive Systemic Sclerosis," *Journal of Rheumatology* 18, no. 8 (1991): 1196–1198.

18. I. Katayana et al., "Topical D₃ (Tacalcitol) for Steroid Resistant Prurigo," *British Journal of Dermatology* 135 (1996): 237–240.

19. T. Acki et al., "1-A, 24-Dihydroxyvitamin D (Tacalcitol) Is Effective against Hailey-Hailey Disease both in Vivo and in Vitro," *British Journal of Dermatology* 139 (1998): 897–901.

Chapter 23

1. June K. Robinson, MD, "Sun Exposure, Sun Protection, and Vitamin D," *JAMA* 294, no. 12 (September 28, 2005): 1541–1543.

2. E. Thieden et al., "Sunscreen Use Related to UV Exposure: Age, Sex and Occupation Based on Personal Behavior Dosimeter Readings and Sun Exposure Behavior Diaries," *Archives of Dermatology* 141 (2005): 967–973.

3. A. Dupuy et al., "Randomized Controlled Trial Testing the Impact of High Protection Sunscreens on Sun Exposure Behavior," *Archives of Dermatology* 141 (2005): 950–956.

4. James Grote, MD, "Vitamin D Deficiency," *JAMA* 295, no. 9 (March 1, 2006): 1002.

5. Jane Higdon, PhD, "Preventing Osteoporosis through Diet and Lifestyle," *The Linus Pauling Institute Research Report* (Spring/Summer 2005): 8–9.

6. Robin Marks, MPH, et al., "The Effects of Regular Sunscreen Use on Vitamin D Levels in an Australian Population," *Archives of Dermatology* 131 (April 1995): 415–421.

7. Michael F. Holick, MD, PhD, "Regular Use of Sunscreen on Vitamin D Levels," *Archives of Dermatology* 131 (November 1995): 1337–1338.

8. Cedric F. Garland, Dr. PH, et al., "Rising Trends in Melanoma: A Hypothesis Concerning Sunscreen Effectiveness," *Annals of Epidemiology* 3, no. 1 (January 1993): 99–102.

Chapter 24

1. Charles B. Clayman, MD (editor), *The American Medical Association Home Medical Encyclopedia* (New York: Random House, 1989), p. 977.

2. "Vitamin D Metabolites (25-Hydroxyvitamin D, 24,25-Dihydroxyvitamin D and 1,25-Dihydroxyvitamin D) and Osteocalcin in Beta-Thalassemia," *Acta Pediatrica* 86 (1997): 594–599.

Chapter 25

1. J. Wortsman et al., "Decreased Bioavailability of Vitamin D in Obesity," *American Journal of Clinical Nutrition* 72 (2000): 690–693.

2. Geneviève C. Major et al., "Supplementation with Calcium plus Vitamin D Enhances the Beneficial Effect of Weight Loss on Plasma Lipid and Lipoprotein Concentrations," *American Journal of Clinical Nutrition* 85 (2007): 54–59.

3. M. A. Pereira et al., "Dairy Consumption, Obesity, and the Insulin Resistance Syndrome in Young Adults: The CARDIA Study," *JAMA* 287 (2002): 2081–2089.

4. K. F. Eriksson et al., "Prevention of Type 2 (Non-Insulin Dependent) Diabetes Mellitus by Diet and Physical Exercise: The 6-Year Malmo Feasibility Study," *Diabetologia* 34 (1991): 891–898.

5. W. C. Knowler et al., "Reduction in the Incidence of Type 2 Diabetes with Lifestyle Intervention or Metformin," *New England Journal of Medicine* 346 (2002): 393–402.

Chapter 26

1. Reinhold Vieth, PhD, "Vitamin D Supplementation, 25-Hydroxyvitamin D Concentrations, and Safety," *American Journal of Clinical Nutrition* 69 (1999): 842–856.

2. John N. Hathcock, PhD, et al., "Risk Assessment for Vitamin D," *American Journal of Clinical Nutrition* 85 (2007): 6–18.

3. John N. Hathcock, PhD, *Vitamin and Mineral Safety* (Washington, D.C.: Council for Responsible Nutrition, 1977), pp. 28ff.

4. D. R. Miller and K. C. Hayes, "Vitamin Excess and Toxicity," in *Nutritional Technology,* vol. 1, J. N. Hathcock, editor (New York: Academic Press, 1982), pp. 81–133.

Index

About the Author

A former editor of *Better Nutrition, GreatLife,* and *Let's Live* (UK) magazines, Frank Murray is the author and/or coauthor of fifty books on health and nutrition, including *100 Super Supplements for a Longer Life* (McGraw-Hill), available in English and Chinese; and *Natural Supplements for Diabetes; Health Benefits Derived from Sweet Orange; Ampalaya: Nature's Remedy for Type 1 and Type 2 Diabetes;* and *How to Prevent Prostate Problems,* all published by Basic Health Publications. A member of the New York Academy of Sciences, the author lives in New York.